If Not Now, WHEN?

Your Path to Wellness

Lupe Silva

7/16/22

Sharon —
Our Health
is our Wealth!
♡ Lupe Silva
Wellness Coach

If Not Now, WHEN?

Your Path to Wellness

Lupe Silva

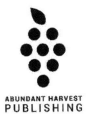

ABUNDANT HARVEST
PUBLISHING

If Not Now, When?
Copyright © 2022 by Lupe Silva

Editing / Formatting: Erik V. Sahakian
Cover Design/Layout: Andrew Enos

Library of Congress Control Number: 2022908368

ISBN 978-1-958137-06-2
First Printing: June 2022

FOR INFORMATION CONTACT:

Abundant Harvest Publishing
www.abundantharvestpublishing.com

Printed in the United States of America

Dedication

I dedicate this book to:

Oscar Sr. (aka BigO), my junior high school sweetheart, my husband, best friend, the greatest father to our sons, and my laughter medicine. Thank you for loving me as much as you do and for being there every step of my life; you always inspire me to be better. Looking forward to our 40th wedding anniversary and beyond...

My two sons, **Oscar and Estevan**, for often teaching me through the glory and trials of raising a family, making me laugh so much (and partly for some of my gray hair), and especially for being the two souls I ADORE. And to our 32 godchildren who have enriched our lives.

My parents, **Ignacio and Alicia Ruiz**, who are now in heaven, for helping form part of who I am today, for wanting me to always strive to be a better person, for all the things I disagreed with growing up and then found myself doing similarly with my own family, for teaching me the importance of paying it forward, and so much more. Mom (whom I called "Mamacita"), after a 12-year battle with Alzheimer's, in her last days, and although the book was in draft form, gave it her blessing so it can reach and help many people. I'll never forget her gentle smile as she took her last breath...

My sisters, **Hilda, Alicia and Adriana**, for showing me

that while we are so uniquely different, we love, need and help each other in a beautiful way—Love you so much!

My sisters-in-Christ, **Reggie, Linda C., Jessica, Sara, Bertha, Evelyn, Trina, Cindy, Teresa, Janis,** and so many others who have provided much support and encouragement to keep me going.

Gerry Warkentine, who initiated many years ago a Bible study group called "Esther's Women of Faith." Thank you so much for your generosity of love, time, and patience which greatly contributed to the realization of this book.

Many friends, mentors, business colleagues, and so many others for helping and encouraging me to share this with the world.

A special thanks to **Dr. Marshall Reddick** for planting the first seeds of natural health, **Dr. Linda Marquez Goodine** for sharing her wellness knowledge, **Ms. Ivy Irvine Bridge** who taught me about iridology, the importance of gut health, and wisdom to help others heal themselves.

And to all my Readers, may this book be a source of inspiration to want to love yourself more and make the decision to take better care of YOU, improve your health, and be happy not just occasionally but **every day**, regardless of circumstances.

Most importantly, I thank God for giving me such an abundance of blessings, challenges to help me grow in His wisdom, answered prayers, and daily guidance to help spread YOUR good news of LOVE and salvation.

Special Dedication

To my dear Ruth Ratican…

"Ruthie," you were the first person I shared my thought about writing a natural health book. Without hesitation, you jumped in and said, "We need to get this kind of message out there and I'll be your editor!"

While you are not here today, I know you are smiling happily from heaven at this accomplishment. You were an amazing lady, friend, wife, and mother of four great children, who I know still miss you dearly.

Until we meet again, my friend…

Disclaimers

It is the author's opinion, as a result of experience and research, that "You are what you think, eat, absorb, eliminate, move (exercise), and sleep." This book is written with the intention to re-teach simple principles that can help you improve your health. It is not intended to diagnose, treat, cure, or heal any illness or ailment. It does not suggest that you stop taking any prescription drugs without consulting with your attending physician.

Take Credit for Your Personal Work

It is the author's recommendation that YOU take credit for any improvement in your overall happiness and health, as a result of your decisions and efforts. You deserve all of the progress and improved conditions you achieve, and more.

Readers This Book Is Written For

This book is written in very basic terms and geared to those who are beginning a more natural or holistic lifestyle. It is not meant to offend anyone who is further along in their understanding or practice of natural health concepts and lifestyles. Further, I've realized over the years of trying so many plans (omnivore, vegetarian, low-fat, high-fat, juice fast, etc.), and as new research develops, I adjust my views and recommendations accordingly. Food trends come and go, however, general nutrition principles remain.

Source Material

You will not find at the end of this book a list of research papers, data, expert testimonials, documentation, studies, or any source references. This book's material and recommendations are a result of the author's personal readings, research, and self-transformation.

Contents

Introduction

Are you sick and tired of being sick and tired? If yes, I'm sorry you are at that point. The good news is that YOU can change and improve your life once and for all. Please know that if someone says it takes a pill, a surgery, one treatment, no exercise needed, or overnight results...**they are lying**. There is **NO** simple solution to this big problem. Start by acknowledging you have hit rock bottom and are ready to transform yourself to live a healthier and happier life, regardless of circumstances.

As the author of a wellness book, I can tell you that I walked the path of being heavy, unhealthy, and unhappy for a long time, so I know firsthand what this means. I was an obese child pretty much until high school when I fell in love and knew it was the weight that was the underlying reason for so much bitterness. Yo yo dieting, stressed to the max in today's overwhelming society, entering menopause at the age of 35, and taking several prescription drugs was enough to push anybody over the edge. Thank you, God, for redirecting my path and finding solutions to health the natural way, changing my perspective, and most of all finding a decent balance in a purpose-filled life.

The primary concept that I found brought more success to myself and others long-term is to concentrate on improving your overall health, not weight loss. When this is done, weight reduction comes naturally.

Thank you for reading this book which will help improve your life in many ways and help you transition from this fast-paced, chemical-ridden world into a more holistic lifestyle that will bring you back to good health, peace, and LOVE.

I've heard there are only two guarantees in life: death and taxes. I can't help you on taxes, so let's do the right thing and pay what is owed. I can't help on the death part either, as we all have our day when we will be called; however, we can make the most of each day by contributing to our best possible health.

This book was written for the average person that has health, weight issues, and is ready and willing to finally make that "change" in lifestyle to reach a new level of health and happiness. Why health and happiness together? Think about it...if your health suffers, are you really happy?

1

What the Heck is Mind Nourishment?

If not now...*WHEN?* Thank you for allowing your curiosity about this chapter to peak. It took me many years to "fix my health" and I'm excited for you that it's now YOUR turn!

Why have you been putting off changing your health, and your life? Is it because you haven't had the time, energy, or self-discipline? Is it because someone has—directly or indirectly—influenced you to stay sick, stressed, or overweight? Have you made intentions to lose weight, or strengthen your body, or increase your flexibility, but somehow never seem to get going, or get very far?

Have you told yourself that you'll start as soon as: your child graduates or moves out, you move to a new home, start your new job, complete your schooling, recover from childbirth, return from vacation, or begin your retirement? Somehow, there's never been enough time.

So, when will you have the time? When you can no longer kneel down to pick up your child? When your last hair falls out? When your relationship ends? When your medical and prescription expenses cost more than your food? When your current stress level puts you out of commission? When you get a diagnosis of a serious condition? When you have a heart attack? When you're dead?

If not now...*WHEN?* If these words stopped you in your tracks and stared you in the face, then this book came to you at this time of your life for a reason. Finding it in the palm of your hand is not some random circumstance. You called it in. You are ready. Your time is now. There is no other time. You are one day away from a life-changing event. It's up to you. The fate of your future is in your hands. You're ready. *You've made up your mind that it's your time. So, it is.*

But how do you do it? How do you get WELL and stay WELL?

You already began the process. *It started in your mind.*

The mind is a powerful thing, a prized possession, for positive or negative. But just like a car, it will perform only what it is programmed to perform, and nothing more. *Programmed?* Cars are programmed, through the input of computerized systems, design, and parts, to perform certain functions at certain levels, on the condition that they are *nourished and cared for* with appropriate fuel and proper maintenance.

Like cars, we are programmed with input. Our beliefs about ourselves and the world, our beliefs about what we should do, think, say, be, and believe are a result of external programming, or conditioning. But reconditioning our minds, and changing our programming, is not only an internal ability, but a responsibility. Our performance depends on it.

What does a car need to run efficiently, smoothly, quickly, and accurately? It needs cleaning and maintenance of both the internal and external parts, checkups, deep cleaning, and tune-ups. And what are the two most basic items a car needs? It needs clean, new, high level fuel and fluids. If it's a battery operated car, it needs to be plugged in to get fully charged, or it's not going to take you anywhere! Lastly, it needs a fully functioning, up-to-date electrical operating system and tires.

Our mind is the operating system of our body. What are we putting into our operating system? Outdated data, negative thoughts, and self-sabotaging beliefs? Or fresh data, positive thoughts, and self-valuing beliefs? Our minds can run rampant, or fall into default patterns, compelling us to run for help, or run around the hamster wheel.

Or, our minds can expand our abilities and exhilarate our experience of being alive.

If we damage or wear out our car, we can buy a new one. We **cannot** buy a new body. *If you wear out your body, how are you going to live?*

What does our mind need to run efficiently, smoothly, quickly, and accurately? Many ingredients are needed to nourish our mind and make it, not only sustainable, but sharp, quick, and powerful. To do that, we want to remove outdated programming and input new programming for our well-being.

Becoming a Master

Each of us is so unique. "One size *cannot* fit all." Know your body and become the master of its strengths, abilities, and assets. Get to know your mind and body by listening closely to how your mind and body respond to specific thoughts, people, foods, tasks, movements, and situations.

Ask your body what it needs:

- to be highly nourished

- to move freely

- to rest and relax

- to be energized and revitalized

- to be strong

- to think clearly and quickly

- to make good judgments and decisions

- to be happy, positive, and excited

Also, ask it what it does NOT need; what thoughts, people, foods, tasks, movements, and situations have the opposite effect. It's very helpful to keep a journal. Every time you get a headache, cold, heartburn, allergy, gas, asthma, tummy ache, cough, bloating, throat mucus, fatigue, sleepiness, irritability, anxiousness, or depressed, write it down and include what you just ate, drank, and who you saw/what you did or experienced right before. Eventually, you will begin to remember and notice trends and therefore make the choices that cause you to feel better, that make you feel your best.

But sometimes, when that task seems to be too challenging, it's helpful to understand the complexity of the mind and its two levels and functions.

Conscious and Subconscious Choices

We have two mind levels: our conscious mind and our subconscious mind. Each has a set of functions and purposes.

Conscious mind:

- Uses logic, deduction, and reason to conclude and make decisions
- Concludes and makes decisions based on the information you feed it
- You must close the door of your conscious mind on every thought of worry, fear, or failure

Subconscious mind:

- Influences the conscious mind
- Primary purpose is to achieve what has been given
- If you do not give your subconscious mind any goals to reach or problems to solve, it will never work for you

- If not, your subconscious mind takes instructions and then acts on them (example: someone tells you, "You look sick." You will probably soon become ill)

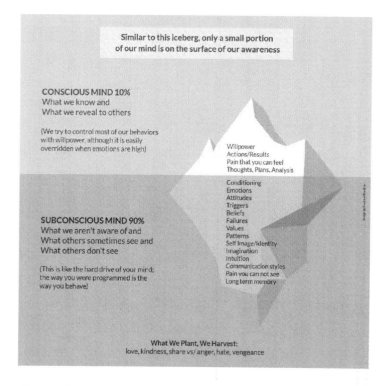

Our subconscious mind stores all that we have been programmed to believe and think about ourselves, and about life. Our conscious mind takes in present data and input, processes it, determines or evaluates it, and responds. But, it does so based on former calculations and evaluations downloaded into the subconscious from all like experiences. In order to change our conscious thinking, beliefs, and actions, we must change the programming of our subconscious mind by inputting new thoughts and beliefs, and releasing outdated versions that are no longer true or valuable for our survival and the person we want to be. Our subconscious mind has infinite abilities, which respond to mental and emotional practices such as visualization, verbally recited affirmations, and positive thinking.

Vision Boards, Visualizations, Affirmations

Input one or more of these into your daily or weekly regimen:

Create a Vision Board: This may sound silly to you. You may be thinking, *I don't have time for that nonsense*, but once you take the time to understand the principle of vision boards and actually create one, you'll find it fun, enlightening, and truly effective. There is plenty of evidence to support that this exercise is highly effective in helping you reach your dreams and goals.

Place your board somewhere that you can see it often, like on a wall near your desk. It doesn't have to be a massive display that everyone sees when they walk in to your space. I have mine on the floor against the wall, but where I can clearly see it.

This is a project you may want to do with a friend, partner, or group. So, set a date and time, invite a few friends, gather some magazines, or download pictures, and make it fun and creative. The magic will make you a believer.

Visualize: You probably have a notion of your favorite

car. You think about it and visualize it often. When you see it on the street, you smile, because seeing what you desire pleases you, and you feel good hoping that you'll be driving it someday.

Close your eyes and picture your *ideal look*...a healthy, vibrant, stronger, happier you. Take it one step further and envision feeling so much better that you are able to help others more, bending over easily and getting up easily, with no more pain, slowness, or loss of balance.

Envision the feeling of these things in your body, and do it often, and you'll be inspired to make it happen, right up to your achieved goal.

Recite Affirmations: It's been proven that saying affirmations in front of a mirror is most effective. Make your own, and keep them simple. Three adjectives are a great formula, and simple. So ladies, **whether** your hair and makeup are done, **feel beautiful**, and go for it!

I am Loveable, Loving, and Loved
I am Healthy, Beautiful, and Whole
I am Happy, Healthy, and Successful
I am Reaching my Health Goals
I am Bold, Brave, and Strong
I am Beautiful, Healthy, and Growing in His Grace

Mindset Shift

As we begin to work with these practices and replace unwanted thoughts and beliefs with newly desired ones, we

[22]

create a mental shift. We shift away from beliefs about ourselves as being *patients* or *victims* who are still suffering, hurting, sick, feeble, or dependent on someone to take care of us. These former self-beliefs are replaced with self-empowering beliefs which lead to creating our own solutions, support, and recovery. We soon realize that *we*, not the doctor, are the source of our own medicine. We realize that we are in charge of our lives and our well-being.

So, how do we integrate outside health advisors into our self-care? Are we no longer to seek a doctor's guidance? Try this mental-verbal shift: "*I'm under my own care*, and I am integrating the advice from a knowledgeable doctor who I feel good about and trust." Please don't misunderstand and think I am saying we don't need doctors. Most are fine human beings living their purpose of helping better their patients, but the responsibility begins with *us.*

I once heard about a study conducted by a hospital doctor who began calling his patients 'clients.' Not surprisingly, there was an overall improvement in his 'client' base, as opposed to his 'patient' base.

Change your thinking and change your life.

Prayer and Meditation

We don't have to be on our knees, sitting in church, holding our thumb and index finger together, or in a pretzel pose, to pray or meditate. We can connect with our higher power whenever, however, and wherever we choose to. It can be challenging to quiet our minds, however.

Try counting backward from **twenty to one**. This really helps. Or, let's focus on *seeing* or *feeling* our breath as it comes in, and follow it as it flows through and out of us. Or, pick a phrase or two words that we say or think to ourselves at each inhale and exhale. Even something as simple as saying, "in" as we inhale and "out" as we exhale, for anywhere from a minute to 10 minutes will do wonders to bring ourselves to a state of calm, peace, centering, and relaxation.

All of these can be done at work, at home, on the sporting field, in the store, at church, at the park, on the front lawn, in the pool, or anywhere. When the mind wanders, just begin again. Don't judge, criticize, or get mad at yourself. Just begin again and continue until you feel good, or for as long as you are able to.

In a *Longevity Now Conference*, David Wolfe said, "You are not a victim of your biology, but a victim of your programming." Contrary to what most of us have been taught, you get to decide what each day will be like for you. Not your biology, not your genes, not your kids, not your parents, and not your past decisions.

When you wake up in the morning, lay still with your eyes closed. Don't get up right away. Feel the quiet of the room, the feel of the soft comfy bed you're nested in, the way the sheets, blanket, and pillow feel on your body. Stretch your body and breathe deeply. With a smile on your face, think about the blessing of this new day and that you get to start in a new way.

Each day is a new chance to begin again. Each day is the holder of a surprise. Expect something good to happen. Well-being is your destiny. Wellness is your birthright. Your belief in these truths is the key to experiencing them. You are always on the journey.

Laughter

Hippocrates was right. Food is the best medicine. But laughter is a close second. Science has shown that laughter releases the "feel good" hormone, endorphins. So, who are you laughing with? When was the last time you laughed? If you can't remember, maybe you've been too focused on working your way through life. Maybe you've been too serious. Maybe you need to laugh at yourself!

When was the last time you did something silly or goofy and laughed at yourself, or laughed out of pure joy?! If we're not laughing, and I mean truly laughing from our belly, then we're decreasing our well-being and joy.

Lucille Ball and Robin Williams are two of my all-time faves that make me laugh every time, no fail. If you need some help transitioning from serious and tense, to relaxed and ready, then turn on some old *I Love Lucy*, or your favorite funny show. And did you know that laughter is a mini abdominal work out? Laugh! The more the better.

Hugs

A student from my Wow! Program (Working on Wellness) once told me, "I don't do hugs unless the person is a family member." A few weeks later, after seeing so much improvement in herself, she opened her arms and offered a big hug to me. I embraced her, and felt the sincere joy for life in her hug. It is experiences like these that have provided me with so many personal rewards affirm my belief that improving our health is vital to living a happy life. Hugs can attribute substantial benefits to our physical and mental well-being.

The Pursuit of Happiness

The happiest of people don't necessarily have the best of everything; they just **make the most of everything**. Happy people are grateful, and grateful people are happy. Interestingly, our Founding Fathers agreed. One of the most important documents in American history, the Declaration of Independence, reads:

> "We hold these truths to be self-evident, that all Men are created equal, that they are endowed by their Creator with certain unalienable Rights, that among these are Life, Liberty, and the Pursuit of Happiness."

So what is happiness, really? No doubt, each of you has your personal definition. I believe health is one of the underlying foundations for happiness, and that if health is not present, it will be difficult, if not impossible, to ever achieve that state of being happy.

Think about it. If you don't have your health, what do you

really have? Unfortunately, as I personally discovered, you don't realize the significance in your life of anything you experience, until you no longer experience it.

The US is among the highest nations of people going to psychologists and psychiatrists than any other nation, yet mental illness is still rising. Our teenage generation has so many material goods (especially technology gadgets), yet suicide rates are at an all-time high.

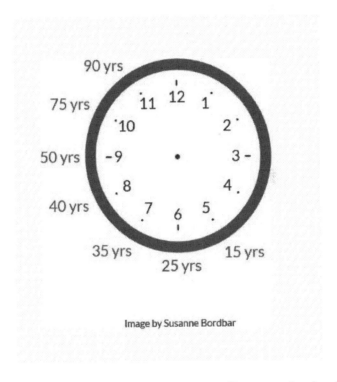

Image by Susanne Bordbar

This visual, though alarming, offers a fascinating perspective of seeing how fast time appears to "fly" and a reminder to all of us to focus on the present moment, appreciating where we are in our journey, and being grateful of life and our window to create optimal health and happiness.

We have, unfortunately, been conditioned to believe that we must *push* and *accomplish, compete and perform, possess and attain, prove and please* in order to live happy and successful lives. We run around in circles, rushing here and there, and everywhere, jumping through never-ending hoops, trying to fill ourselves up with external approval, acceptance, and things, in the belief that we will soon accomplish enough to finally reach that status of happiness.

We gather and collect possessions, clothes, beauty aids, products, toys, money, friends, and fans, expecting to receive the gift of peace and happiness. "When I get a bigger house, a new car, married, a relationship, money in the bank, thin..." The quest just leaves us exhausted, insecure, and emptier than before we began the search. And, completing one accomplishment, or acquiring one possession, only leads to the search for the next one.

Happiness doesn't have a price tag. We can't buy it. It's not a final destination that we will arrive at some day. Not even with our MasterCard! Happiness is a state of mind that only we can create, a state we create within ourselves. You've heard the definition of insanity, right? "Insanity is repeatedly doing the same thing the same way, and expecting a different result." If you want to be happy, you need to do things differently, look at things differently. True, deep, sustainable happiness is more fulfilling than any person, thing, or experience can give you. And it comes without a hefty monthly bill! As humans, we will never reach a destination of perfection, but we can experience happiness. In reading this book, you are already on that path.

Health and happiness are inextricably linked. The better you nourish yourself, the better you feel and the bigger the impact you can have on the world. In a transformed world, everyone is doing work they love and are easily and abundantly compensated financially and spiritually for it.

Negative Thoughts, Attitude, Energy

Surprising to most people is the truth that negativity is a state that we've been trained to be in. What?! Now, don't start looking to blame all the people in your life who ever taught you, or caused you to learn how to be negative. That won't end well. Most likely, they weren't even aware they were doing it.

So, let's start from a new vantage point. Without analyzing yourself or criticizing yourself for falling into that habit, instead, ponder this: If you could replace a negative viewpoint, thought, statement, belief, or emotion with a positive one, how would you do that? What would that look like? Well, it would feel better. It would possibly feel a bit awkward at first because you're so accustomed to falling into that harmless gossip, agreeing with someone about something because you care about commiserating with them, or stating the "reality." Deep inside of you, in your gut, in your heart, and in your head, none of those really ever felt good to you, right?

So, what if you looked for something to point out or think about that made you feel good? Something that you appreciate? A beautiful flower, the warm sun on your body after being cold, the cute face of your pet as it nuzzles you, the flock of birds flying and dipping in the blue sky, or the kindness of a total stranger yesterday. What if you made it a point to look for those things to think about, point out, and appreciate every day? What if you changed the subject when your friend, partner, family member, or co-worker started talking in the negative? What if you redirected them to something that you know they would appreciate, marvel, or smile at?

You can retrain your mind to focus on positive, loving, beautiful, happy things. And the best part of this is that you will begin to notice those positive thoughts, things, people, and experiences start happening for you more and more every day. And your energy will change. Your body will change. Your mind will change. You will change into a new you that you really feel good about.

Purpose—Your BIG "WHY"

What is my purpose for teaching wellness? That goes back to my why. I described my transformation in the introduction, but to summarize, I was overweight, unhealthy, and unhappy for many years. I was an obese child until high school, when I realized that my carrying so much excess weight was the underlying reason for so much bitterness in my heart. As a result of carrying that weight, my knees hurt all the time. I was diagnosed with rheumatoid arthritis in high school. Yo yo dieting into adulthood and stressed to the max from trying to keep up with what was expected of me, I entered menopause at age 35. I took five prescription drugs, including Prozac for depression, anti-inflammatory drugs, hormone meds, sleeping pills, etc. I had insomnia and so the next day I had to drink five cups of coffee in order to function and be productive to keep myself from dragging and falling asleep.

The deeper I went into ill health and chemical dependency, the more attention, care, and concern I got from loved ones. So I craved ailments. Though no one told me, nor did I have a clue, my bad habits and poor health drained my adrenals. I was literally falling apart.

I was in my forties, working with Marshal Reddick, who was always happy and healthy, when I understood the real reason he had never been to a doctor or a hospital in his life. He had always eaten pretty healthy and had an extraordinarily positive mindset. I put those two cause and effect elements together in my mind, and I knew I could do it too. That connection was powerful motivation that inspired me to change my life in a big way. After being sick and tired of being sick and tired, I began my transformation. And I have never looked back.

Why are you making the decision to change your life right now? There has to be a powerful drive behind it. **A powerful why** is a critical component in our transformation. If your why is not strong enough, powerful enough, or defined enough, you will NOT have the desire, drive, discipline, or inspiration to be committed to the shift necessary to embrace change and transform into a better you.

Final Thoughts

A child is born with only two fears: falling and loud noises. This makes sense when you think of the trip down the birth canal out into a world of noise. All other fears have been taught to the child as they grow up. As a result of all we are taught throughout our lives, we develop two new and unnatural fears: fear of failure or loss, and fear of criticism or rejection.

Fear of failure is the primary cause for failure in adulthood. Fear of criticism holds us back, undermines our confidence, and destroys our desire to create our own happiness because we are afraid of displeasing others, disappointing others, and not being approved by others.

Knowledge is power, but **wisdom is life giving**. We have seen an increase in information and knowledge, but a decrease in wisdom. Wisdom is knowing what is true for you, listening to your own mind and body, and doing what is true for you, not following what others have told you is true for you. Wisdom is knowing that being true to your purpose and needs is the path to your peace, health, and happiness.

Albert Einstein, one of the greatest minds in history, said, "Unless you make changes, you will have the same results,"

…anything else is just INSANITY!

Is it time to release your fears? Is it time to please yourself? Is it time to care about approving and loving yourself? If you answered no, or you're not sure, then take some time to ask your inner self, why not? Why did you start to become afraid to please yourself? It's your choice. Fear of failure and fear of criticism are not your natural state. Is it time to get off the hamster wheel? Is it time to stop doing the same thing and accepting the same result? If yes, then you are going to so love yourself and your results. That is the power of Mind Nourishment.

2

What Are Nature's Nutrients?
Air, Water, Earth, and Sun

Air and Breath

It is the first breath that begins life and the last breath that ends life. While we can survive without food for one to two months and water for three to seven days, we can survive without air for no more than three minutes. Breath is our most essential connection to life. A human takes an average of over 20,000 breaths a day. When we stop to think about it, we understand how profound breath is.

Breath can be one of the most vital factors influencing our state of mind which, in turn, affects our physical health and well-being. Knowing this, it is an interesting phenomenon that most people do not breathe properly. This may come as a shock, especially since many of us consider breathing, automatic and natural. However, the lack of breathing properly eventually causes our health to deteriorate, which shows up in symptoms such as higher stress levels, energy loss, and even weight gain.

Like our heartbeat, the rate at which we breathe can be measured. This is known as the "respiratory rate," referring to the expected amount of breaths inhaled while we are at rest. Of course, these rates differ based on lung volume, body size, etc., but the ideal rate is between 12 and 20 breaths per minute. Many of us do not breathe within the ideal range, which is one of the common detriments to our health. Breathing through our lungs, instead of our belly and diaphragm, is another.

There are several specific components of efficient, body-rejuvenating breathing. It is challenging to accurately and sufficiently describe them here, but due to breath's priority in our vitality, I highly recommend breath work classes where breathing techniques are integrated into the class. These classes are a beautiful, highly worthwhile investment in our health.

Most of us sit hunched over all day, whether over a computer, crafting or hobby, job activity, steering wheel, smart phone, video games, or television. Too much time in a permanent forward stance puts excess pressure and repetitive stress on the cervical spine, shoulders, and neck. Additionally, this position cuts airflow supply, as the diaphragm constantly compresses the ribs, causing shorter and shallower breathing. Then we wonder why we are drained of energy by the end of the day. If we make it a point to get up to stretch our backs, shoulders, and neck every half hour or hour, we will feel the difference during the day, as well as at the end of the day.

Stress contributes to improper breathing, but the reverse is also true. Inefficient breathing can increase our stress levels.

When we are stressed, our breaths become quicker, shallower, and shorter, which increases the stress.

After our prayer of appreciation, our Wow! Program classes always start with deep breathing exercises, to set us in the right frame of mind, body, and spirit. Deep breathing is a practice that produces amazing benefits including acting as a natural tranquilizer, increasing oxygen intake, increasing serotonin levels, eliminating damaging toxins, reducing heart and respiratory rates, reducing blood pressure, enhancing our mood, centering and grounding us, and more.

I recommend the following quick deep breathing exercise as often as possible, especially first thing in the morning when the air is cleaner and there is less environmental pollution than during the evening hours. This lowers stress, reduces anxiety, relieves negativity, and calms our busy distracted mind.

- If possible, stand up. If not, sit up straight. Close your eyes.

- Take a deep breath and hold it when you have reached your lung capacity. (Note: you should inhale twice as fast as you exhale.)

- Then, very slowly, release your breath through your teeth without opening your mouth.

- Do this as many times as you wish to feel immediate results and a calmer state.

Interestingly, in my many past efforts to lose weight, I kept an article from February 2001 in my exercise file, "Breathing is Better than Exercise." Author, C.J. Fischer, explains that you can lose weight the "Oxycise!" way—a simple 15 minute daily series of deep breathing exercises done while stretching and holding the body in certain positions. Using only this process, she lost 45 pounds in six months, with no big changes in her food intake. The importance of breathing properly and in developing a breathing exercise practice, to reach optimal health, cannot be overemphasized.

Water

I find it fascinating that water is referenced in the Bible 722 times. Our bodies are made up of approximately 70% water and, as such, water is the liquid of choice for the body's optimal health. Recent studies show that 75% of Americans may suffer from chronic dehydration, which causes emotional sensitivity, nausea, high blood pressure, kidney disease, and hundreds of other serious and even life-threatening conditions. I've seen so many times with students who have headaches, kidney trouble, and tons of other random concerns that by merely increasing their daily water consumption, their condition improves.

For years, I heard the common recommendation, "Drink eight glasses of water per day." Think about that. Does it make sense for a seven-year old child, whose average weight is 60 pounds, and a 300-pound adult to drink the same amount of water each day? Definitely not. A better recommendation is to drink half your body weight in ounces of water each day. With this dosage a 150-pound person would drink 75 ounces of water per day, approximately nine and a half glasses, and a 60-pound child would drink 30 ounces of water per day, or approximately three and a half glasses. It may seem like a lot of water, but it's a habit that becomes routine.

To fill that requirement and keep you within a healthy regimen, it's best to stay away from most other drinks. During colder weather months, you probably will not crave as much water as in the summer, so be creative. Drink hot lemon water and use good judgement on your body's water needs.

We often mistake thirst for hunger. If given an opportunity to absorb a glass of water for a few minutes before automatically reaching for food, your body would let you know that you were really just thirsty, and the food craving was only a means of satisfying an emotional need, or boredom, or just a habit.

Today, there are hundreds, if not thousands, of choices of water, including new trends of "infused" water and lightly flavored water. Some are great, but most are not. Don't be fooled. Read the label carefully. Once you start seeing "natural flavors" in the ingredients, put it down. That typically is a label to cover up chemicals. Get back to basics and just throw in a slice of lemon, lime, strawberry, mint, cucumber, celery, or any other fruit, vegetable, or herb that appeals to you, and you just made your own infused drink.

You lose water through urination, respiration, and sweating, and you lose more water when you're active than when you're sedentary. Diuretics, such as caffeine pills, certain medications, and alcohol may increase the amount of water your body absorbs from your skin, muscles, tissue, and organs. A strong odor in your urine, along with a yellow or amber color, may be an indication that you are not getting enough water. But, note that riboflavin, a B vitamin, and dietary supplements that contain large amounts of riboflavin, will also make your urine bright yellow. Certain medications can also change the color of urine. These and other causes increase your need to replenish through water content foods and beverages, to bring your body back to balance.

There are so many benefits of water, the most important of which is maintaining sufficient hydration keeps you from dying. Yikes! Add to that better skin, less constipation, increased mental clarity, less puffiness and bloating, better sleep, more energy, less irritability and moodiness, improved performance, and decreased joint pain. I think you get my point. Just drink more water!

Avoiding fluoride in your water—and your toothpaste—is highly recommended. This may come as a surprise to you as it did to me. I grew up going to the dentist twice a year for cleanings and fluoride applications. After studying—and personally researching this because I couldn't believe it—I confirmed how toxic fluoride really is. I've avoided it ever since. Trust me on this, or do your own research.

According to a 2016 article, author Jon Levine reports,

"You've been drinking water wrong—this is how to do it, according to Chinese medicine." Drinking cold or iced water might invite "a chorus of criticism," wrote Nicole Liu, a self-described "devoted hot water drinker," in her article for the Los Angeles Times. When it comes to health, traditional Chinese medicine promotes "harmony." It is believed that drinking cold water takes the body out of equilibrium by knocking it out of its optimal working temperature.

"In regards to the body, cold blocks the meridian channels, slows—and even congeals—blood circulation, and diminishes organ functioning to less than optimal ability," said Mee Lain Ling, a registered doctor of traditional Chinese medicine, on her website.

Room temperature water is best for the body. Only on very hot days do I enjoy drinking ice-cold water. You may have heard that "shocking" your body with ice-cold water helps speed up a slow metabolism, but this is not true. You've always known it. With symptoms like brain freeze and toothaches, your body is telling you that ice-cold beverages are hard for your sensitive body. On occasion it's okay, but make your norm room temperature. Your body is a sensitive instrument. Shocking it affects its natural sensitivity.

The quality of water you drink is also extremely important. Consider using glass containers to drink your water as metal, plastic, Styrofoam, and even paper products contain chemicals that are toxic to the body. I highly recommend you invest in a water filter system. Yes, alkaline water is wonderful; however, I prefer a balanced mix of 80-90%

alkaline and the rest spring water. We invested in a PristineHydro WATER REVIVAL SYSTEM for our home that produces structured, 100% acid free, chemical free, fluoride free, high alkaline (mineralized with a high magnesium bicarbonate content) water. We use it for drinking water, good quality ice cubes, rinsing all our produce, cooking food, and general food preparation. We love it.

Earthing

Earthing may be a new word in your vocabulary. My computer didn't even recognize it and marked it as misspelled. Earthing is a means of connecting us back to nature, the ultimate source of health and healing, done by walking barefoot, playing with your hands, or laying bare-skinned in the dirt, garden soil, grass, or sand. It's that simple, nothing "hokey" about it. It's all scientifically proven. In fact, I'm a true testimonial! I've been earthing for some time now. I've changed my earthing area from my front lawn to my back lawn, in case some of my neighbors thought I was crazy walking barefoot on our moist front lawn in my pj's at the crack of dawn. Just kidding. I changed to my backyard because we have a lot more grass there.

We used to live near a small park. Every other day, I'd see a little Asian gal who appeared to be earthing. After I saw her the first few times, I had to ask if she was earthing. With a sweet smile, she confirmed she was 83 years old and had a regular practice of grounding for one hour. Sometimes, she went to the volleyball sand area and walked barefoot there. She ended her trip to the park by picking up weeds and any trash she encountered. "It's my way of helping the earth." What a beautiful way of contributing to the world.

My "girls," Zoe and Ruby (my four-pound dogs), innately love to roll around and sunbathe in our flowerbeds and lawns. Kids innately love to take off their shoes and run barefooted. Most of us used to play in the dirt, run in the grass, swim in the ocean, walk on the sand, dig in the soil, or just walk barefoot on the sidewalk. Remember how wonderful it felt? Why? Earthing is the most natural and safe way to improve your health and sense of happiness. I read an article about how landscapers and gardeners have less health afflictions. They work every day with soil, grass, and live plants.

It's so simple, yet astoundingly profound. Earthing is not a treatment. It is a missing link in the health equation, a foolproof method of returning to your core and connecting with nature in a way that we've nearly abandoned. So, go ahead! Take off your shoes, cover your hands with the soil and sand, lay on the grass, and enjoy the warmth or coolness of the earth. Get recharged, recalibrated, and rejuvenated with life's natural energy.

Grounding

As humans, we function by way of our central nervous system, a series of electrical nerve impulses that work miracles. Some individuals who are sick, in pain, or have inflammation might be electron deficient. Others may have an interference in the nerve impulses. You've watched this scene: someone is having a heart attack and paramedics try to revive the person by giving them electrical shocks. Exposure to our precious earth provides "electrical nutrition" in the form of electrons.

However, too much electrical and electromagnetic frequencies from our modern lifestyles have the opposite effect of reviving someone. Earthing is essential for maintaining our body's natural state of well-being, but we can't always do that. Sitting at computers, working with electrical tools and devices, having long phone conversations, watching tv for hours a week, being surrounded by lights, appliances, meters, and electrical currents in every building, and driving electrical cars, our body's electrical system becomes quickly, easily, and many times severely overloaded. This results in nervousness, stress, confusion, fatigue, vision and sensory problems, loss of balance, weakened immune systems, illness, and more.

Preventing ourselves from being shocked, overstimulated, and out of balance during our electrically charged daily habits and environments requires getting "grounded." Grounding is a means of using natural earth elements, or designed manmade elements connected to the earth elements, to diffuse all of the excess electricity and moving it out of our bodies and into the earth, which innately knows what to do with it.

Some grounding methods include:

- a grounding pad under your computer keyboard
- a grounding pad on your work chair
- a floor pad in your workspace
- grounding pillowcases and sheets for your bed
- deep breathing
- showering (water is an earth element covering our skin, our body's largest organ)
- thinking positive thoughts

Earth is nature's original anti-inflammatory and can remedy our deficiencies, improve our central nervous system function, recalibrate and strengthen our immune systems, revive our natural mental, emotional, and physical energy, and optimize our sleep. Here are additional benefits of earthing and grounding:

- rapid reduction of inflammation
- dynamic blood flow improvement to supply and circulate vital oxygen and nutrients
- reduction of stress
- increase in energy
- improvement in sleep
- acceleration of healing from injuries and surgery
- reduction or elimination of chronic pain
- significant sense of well-being

You earth and ground every day when you shower or bathe. It's no coincidence that we come out with great ideas and a sense of renewal.

In wellness conventions I've attended, it has been so exciting and welcoming to walk into a room of 2,000 grounded chairs, each with a small pad on the chair connected to an electrical wire to the ground, grounding and rebalancing us while we sat. Someone not familiar with this science may not understand and be afraid of being electrocuted. Mr. Clinton Ober, co-author of a great book, entitled *Earthing*, created this genius project for us as we sat through the all-day conference.

Here are some comments and reviews by professionals on the book *Earthing*:

"People have lost touch with the Earth. From a biblical perspective, people who lose touch with the Earth lose touch with God. Earthing reconnects us to the planet, to others, and in a sense, to God." – Gabriel Cousens, M.D., author of *Spiritual Nutrition*

"Earthing ranks right up there with the discovery of penicillin. This book is probably the most important health read of the twenty-first century." – Ann Louise Gittleman, PH.D., C.N.S, author of *The Fat Flush Plan*

"Hormonal imbalances are so prevalent among women. Earthing has a profoundly beneficial effect in helping to balance the system and reduce symptoms." – Amanda Ward,

N.D., Encinitas, CA

"Earthing may be as fundamental as sunlight, air, water, and nutrients. 'May the Ground be with you!'" – Gary E. Schwartz, P.H.D., Professor of Psychology and Medicine, University of Arizona

"This works! It has great promise. Something simple that should be used everywhere." – Richard Delany, M.D., Milton, MA

The majority of people want the most health benefits for the least amount of work. Grounding and earthing are it! There is no work, only relaxation, rest, and play.

Sun

Clocks. We have them in practically every room because we want to be constantly reminded of time, to stay on top of our busy schedule. Yet, I remember never seeing one in my grandparents' house in Mexico. Whenever we visited them I was amazed they used the natural sunrise to know what time to wake up—not to mention the church bells and the neighborhood roosters!

Today, people are awakened by an alarm system placed on their nightstand next to their heads. Sadly, I've heard that more and more people use their smartphones as their wake up system. I say "sadly" because most don't know how much electromagnetic radiation cell phones produce and how much this interferes with their sleep and nightly cellular rejuvenation. (I have more on this in Chapter 5.)

You've heard many times that the sun is good for you, but too much sun is bad for you. Yes, and yes. For optimal health, we need "direct sun" medicine, which is best before 10 a.m. and after 4 p.m., "safe sun" time, before and after the strongest rays are in effect. A minimum of 10 minutes a day is beneficial. Be spontaneous and enjoy the light and warmth of the sun every chance you get during the safe hours. And while you are at it, you can work on deep breathing—an additional benefit on your Wellness Path.

A few of the many benefits our sun provides include:

- Mood boost and SAD reduction (Seasonal Affective Disorder, aka the winter blues): People actually smile more in the presence of the sun (depression is heightened by lack of sunlight). This happens as sunshine boosts levels of serotonin, the body's natural happy hormone.

- Relief from aches and pains: The sun warms the body's muscles and eases stiffness, reducing the pain caused by inflammatory conditions, such as arthritis.

- Energy boost: Melatonin, a chemical produced naturally by the body to regulate your sleep is produced less in the summertime. This explains your lesser need for sleep for maintaining energy levels. In addition, being awakened by natural light, rather than the alarm clock, helps infuse you with positivity.

- Skin remedy: Sun exposure can help heal skin

[47]

conditions such as psoriasis, acne, and eczema. Keep "safe sun" hours in mind.

- Fertility boost: The sun reduces the hormone melatonin, which weakens fertility. Thus, it's more likely you'll conceive a child during the summer. Sunlight not only increases your fertility, but it also increases the length of your fertility period. In addition, it boosts testosterone levels in men, making the summer ideal for baby-making.

- Facilitates weight loss: Higher levels of serotonin in the body makes you feel happy, while also suppressing the appetite. You'll eat less during warmer weather.

- Boosts our body's ability to produce vitamin D through the sun's UVB rays on our skin:

  o essential for absorbing calcium to keep your bones healthy

  o helps reduce heart disease and multiple sclerosis

  o eases Irritable Bowel Syndrome

  o helps keep your teeth strong

  o boosts your immune system

  o reduces your risk of several cancers and other serious health conditions

Most people think of vitamin D as the "bone vitamin," but

recent discoveries show that vitamin D is essential for a tremendous number of normal bodily processes. Virtually every tissue type in the body possesses receptors for the activated vitamin D molecule, defining vitamin D as a true hormone. Low vitamin D levels are associated with increased risks of cardiovascular and neurological disease, cancer, diabetes, and autoimmune disorders.

The majority of Americans have vitamin D levels below the minimum recommended. Fortunately, vitamin D supplementation has been shown to be protective for all these conditions, when taken at the dosage of at least 2,000 IU/day. Nutrition and exercise impact the efficacy of this vitamin and other supplements...another reason for "clean eating" and appropriate movement. As with any supplementation, consult with your healthcare provider to ensure you are getting the adequate amount for your body, age, and condition.

So how much sun is enough? How much is too much? Simply living above the 37th parallel (anything above New Mexico) is reported to increase the risk because the days available for UVB production are limited. Additionally, people of color need more time in the sun, since the melanin in their skin acts as a natural sunscreen. Women need more sun exposure than men and, in particular, pregnant women.

Sunscreen

While it's commonly recommended to slather our skin before bathing in the sun, after knowing what's in it, you will understand the reason for my recommendation. How many of us sit or stand in buildings all day, then slather on sunscreen, sunglasses, hats, or protective suits, just to spend time outside. Perhaps this might surprise you, anger you, or even stun you, but for the sake of your health, AVOID sunscreen!

While sunscreens are meant to do just that—put a screen over your skin to protect you—most are loaded with toxins that actually do more harm than good. Harmful parabens have been discovered in nearly all cancerous tumors. Parabens are common ingredients in makeup, shampoo, conditioners, and most sunscreen products! Sunscreen manufacturers don't claim their products prevent skin cancer, only sunburn. With that said, covering the largest organ of your body—your skin—with toxins that easily seep through your skin surface pores and enter your tissue, bones, muscles, blood supply, and cells is not a good idea. Your skin acts like a sponge, so whatever you put on it, it will gobble up. Would you feel comfortable admitting that you eat sunscreen?

In addition to endangering the health of humans, our fish and wildlife are endangered by the presence of sunscreen in our waters and earth. Research reports that one of the common ingredients in sunscreen is known to be toxic to ocean coral, contributing to the decline of reefs around the world. Oxybenzone, a UV-filtering chemical compound found in 3,500 brands of sunscreen worldwide, can be fatal to baby coral and damaging to adults in high concentrations, according to *a study published in the Archives of Environmental Contamination and Toxicology*, with the highest concentrations around coral reefs popular with tourists, particularly those in Hawaii and the Caribbean.

So prevent skin and other cancers by avoiding sunscreen, but be sure to get your small doses of safe sun as often as you can.

A great book to read on the topic of sunscreen is Dr. Elizabeth Plourde's, *Sunscreens: Biohazard, Treat as Hazardous Waste.*

Nature provides all the nutrients the human mind, body, and spirit need to maintain health, prevent disease, balance our modern day stress-filled lifestyles, and thrive. Don't underestimate the power of mother nature as a one-stop elixir. My prescription for you: a daily dose of fresh air, water, earth, and sun.

3

What Are Your Primary Foods?

Relationships, Forgiveness, and Agape Love

Relationships

What do you think is the most important food for humans? Broccoli? Spinach? Kale? Perhaps our drinking water? After all, our body is primarily made up of water. What about our faith?

Just as when I first heard this question, my Wow! Program students answered "yes" to all those items. However, for most human beings, the most important food is the relationships that we develop during our lifetime. Understanding this was one of the most profound shifts I made as a student at IIN (Institute for Integrative Nutrition), the world's largest holistic nutrition school. My appreciation is deep for IIN founder/director, Joshua Rosenthal, for creating such an amazing community of change, to better our world through nutrition.

In his book, *Integrative Nutrition: Feed Your Hunger for Health & Happiness*, he explores the difference between ordinary food and what he calls "primary foods." Primary foods are more than what is on your plate, including healthy relationships. Relationships include the relationships you have with your:

- spirituality/God/religion
- spouse/soulmate
- children
- parents
- grandparents
- friends
- pets
- health
- career
- finances
- palace/environment (home)
- service (pay it forward)
- education
- home cooking
- movement/exercise
- fun
- addiction
- yourself (are you happy with you?)

Primary foods can fill your soul and satisfy your hunger for life. **When primary foods are balanced and satisfying, your life feeds you**, making what you eat secondary. Interesting! Can you see why these are considered primary foods? While this may seem trivial to some, it can make a HUGE difference for many of us.

In the hundreds of seminars I've attended with one of my mentors, Dr. Linda, I heard her say, **"We are overfed and undernourished."** This is such a profound statement—not just in food, but in relationships and actions, as well.

We cannot underestimate the importance of friendship, especially the friendships women share with other females. Women connect with each other differently from the way they connect with men, and from the way men connect with men. Women share feelings; whereas men often form relationships around activities. A man rarely sits down with a buddy to talk about how they feel about certain things or how their personal lives are going. Jobs? Yes. Sports? Yes. Cars? Yes. Fishing, hunting, golf? Yes. Feelings? Rarely. But women do it all the time.

Spending time with a friend is just as important to our general health as jogging or working out at a gym. Women provide support systems that help each other to deal with stress and difficult life experiences. We share from our souls and, evidently, that is very good for our health. The physical benefit of quality "girlfriend time" is that it generates more serotonin, a neurotransmitter that helps combat depression and can create a general feeling of well-being.

Finances, health, and relationships are constantly under strain, and are a main concern for so many. Regular feelings of resentment, jealousy, and hatred put us in a negative state. Wherever you go and whatever you do, always look to see how you can help and give what you can. We get what we put out. Look at other people through the lens of love.

(At the end of this chapter you will find an exercise that may help you better understand the balance in your "circle of life".)

The visual extension of what you just learned is found in Joshua Rosenthal's book.

Forgiveness: Letting Go

When someone you care about hurts you, you can hold on to anger, resentment, and thoughts of revenge. Or, you can embrace forgiveness and move forward with your life. Nearly everyone has been hurt by the actions or words of another. Perhaps your mother criticized your parenting skills, your coworker wrongly blamed you for the unsuccessful project, or your spouse had an affair. These wounds can leave you with lasting feelings of anger, bitterness, and even vengeance.

Forgiveness can be challenging, especially if the person who hurt you doesn't admit wrong or doesn't speak of their sorrow. Yet, getting another person to change their actions, behavior, or words isn't the point of forgiveness. Think of forgiveness more in terms of how it can change your life—by bringing you peace, happiness, emotional vitality, and spiritual healing. Forgiveness can take away the power the other person continues to consume in your life.

Forgiveness doesn't mean you deny the other person's responsibility for hurting you, and it doesn't minimize or justify the wrong. You can forgive the person without excusing the act. Forgiveness means letting go of the energy, emotion, and focus that you are spending on the person, the grudge, and the wrongful action. Letting go brings back your energy and a kind of peace that helps you go on with life, like setting a prisoner free—but the prisoner is you.

It's easy to hold on to a grudge when you're hurt by someone you love and trust. You may become angry, sad or confused. However, if you dwell on hurtful events or situations, grudges, resentment, vengeance, and hostility can take root. If you allow negative feelings to crowd out positive feelings, you may find yourself swallowed up by your own bitterness or sense of injustice. The effects of holding on to a grudge can be quite harmful. You may pay the price repeatedly by bringing anger and bitterness into every relationship and new experience. Your life might become so wrapped up in the wrong that you can't enjoy the present. You may become depressed or anxious. You even might feel your life lacks meaning or purpose, or that you're at odds with your spiritual beliefs. You might lose valuable and enriching connectedness with others. If you cannot forgive, then you will most likely be the one who pays, by holding on to your own poisonous emotions and gossip.

If you find it difficult to forgive, consider the situation

from the other person's point of view. Ask yourself why they would behave in such a way. Perhaps you would have reacted similarly if you faced the same situation. In addition, consider broadening your view of the world. Expect occasional imperfections from the people in your life. You may want to reflect on times you've hurt others and times when others have forgiven you. It can also be helpful to write in a journal, pray or use guided meditation, or talk with a person you've found to be wise and compassionate, such as a spiritual leader, a mental health provider, or an impartial loved one or friend.

If the hurtful event involved someone whose relationship you otherwise value, forgiveness can lead to reconciliation. This isn't always the case, however. Reconciliation might be impossible if the offender has died or is unwilling to communicate with you. In other cases, reconciliation might not be appropriate. Nonetheless, forgiveness is possible, even if reconciliation isn't.

Forgiveness is a commitment to a process of change. To begin, you might:

- Consider the value of forgiveness and its importance in your life at a given time.
- Reflect on the facts of the situation, how you've reacted, and how this combination has affected your life, health, and well-being.

- When you're ready, actively choose to forgive the person who's offended you.

- Move away from your role as victim and release the control and power the offending person and situation have had in your life.

If you haven't reached a state of forgiveness, being near the person who hurt you might be tense and stressful. To handle these situations, remember you can choose to attend or avoid specific functions and gatherings. Respect yourself and do what seems best. If you choose to attend, don't be surprised by a certain amount of awkwardness and perhaps even more intense feelings. Do your best to keep an open heart and mind. You might find the experience helps you to move forward with forgiveness.

Consider how forgiveness can lead you down the path of physical, emotional, and spiritual well-being. Letting go of grudges and bitterness can make way for compassion, kindness, and peace that can lead to:

- healthier relationships
- greater spiritual and psychological well-being
- less anxiety, stress, and hostility
- lower blood pressure
- reduction in pain
- fewer symptoms of depression
- lower risk of alcohol or substance abuse
- lower risk of relying on medications, overeating, or

eating disorders

What if you are the one who needs forgiveness? The first step is to honestly assess and acknowledge the wrongs you've done and how those wrongs have affected others. At the same time, avoid judging yourself too harshly. We are human and will make mistakes. If you're truly sorry for something you've said or done, consider admitting it to those you've harmed. Speak of your sincere sorrow or regret, and specifically ask for forgiveness—without making excuses.

However, remember you can't force someone to forgive you. Others need to move to forgiveness in their own time. Whatever the outcome, commit to treating others with compassion, empathy, and respect. As you let go of grudges, you'll no longer define your life by how you've been hurt and may even find compassion and understanding. By embracing forgiveness, you can also embrace peace, hope, gratitude, and joy. It's ALL about LOVE!

4

Why Change Fuel?

Why do we need to change our fuel? ***We are overfed and undernourished!*** What fueled our physical-chemical-mental body balance for centuries no longer has the rich and nutrient density to fulfill our needs for optimum health. Our once abundant soil that provided rich fuel (vegetables, fruits, carbohydrates, and plant-based fats and proteins) for us and our livestock has been so overused that its minerals and nutrients are practically depleted. It's true! We have become literally **"dirt poor."**

If our soil is depleted, whatever is grown in it is also depleted. Why is this a big deal? If we decided we could make the gas for our vehicles stretch further if we diluted it with another type of gas, or liquid, and increased that over time, we would soon experience a decline in the function of our cars. Eventually, we would have no functioning cars to take us anywhere. It's a scary thought, if we apply this principle to our bodies, though it is a reality.

Our bodies are designed to run on living vegetables, fruits, plant-based proteins, carbohydrates, fats, and occasional naturally grazing animals, fish, and fowl. As we incrementally "dilute" our natural nutrient-rich diet with choices that aren't nutrient rich, we soon experience a decline in the function of our physical-chemical-mental bodies *and spirit*. In time, we will be unable to think, create, act, or move in the same ways we used to. Taken to an extreme, over time, we will be afflicted with disease and die decades earlier than we should.

To get the same nutritional value that our soil provided two or more hundred years ago, today we need to eat 10 bunches of spinach, compared to one. Who can commit to eating that kind of volume? This doesn't take into consideration the depletion that results from the high amounts of chemical-ridden pesticides and fertilizers that have become the norm to use on soil for increasing the harvest time and volume. Or the depletion that occurs from pollutants and contaminants released into the oceans from industrial and commercial buildings and human negligence, and oceans of water that we recycle to use in our daily lives. Or that which occurs from the injection of artificial hormones into cows, chickens, and turkeys to make them fatter (meatier), or in a continual state of reproducing. Or that resulting from the GMO (genetically modified organisms) processes to our food crops.

Organic vs. Conventional Foods

Conventional foods are just foods that became commonly eaten over a long period of time, for various reasons. Conventional nutritionists advocate the SAD (Standard American Diet). This diet tends to be very acidic and—*based on our nation's current state of health*—has proven ineffective at optimizing health and body function and preventing disease. Even the acronym SAD is not positive. What is appealing about eating a sad diet? (More on the topic of acid in Chapter 7.)

Where did the "milk is good for everyone" commercial go? We were raised with the belief that we need milk for maintaining our bodies' optimum levels of vitamin D. However, D is not a vitamin, and we cannot actually obtain vitamin D from drinking cow milk. It is produced naturally by the body and enhanced by sufficient time in the natural sun.

After learning how cows are raised, fed, and treated, we figured out why milk isn't good for everyone. Today's cow milk is highly homogenized (processed away from natural) and loaded with hormones and antibiotics, which are then passed on to us…especially our growing children. Growing children? Sadly, our children are growing in abnormally high rates toward obesity and disease. "Good mothers" grew up with the belief that milk was the primary survival for their children. In actuality, a child loses the enzyme lactase, which absorbs and processes the lactose in cow milk, between the age of two and three. Add to that the fact that the dairy industry genetically alters cows to increase their pregnancy to produce more milk, then injects them with artificial growth hormones to increase their size, and you've got a recipe for disease and disaster.

Not long ago while teaching a Wow! Program class, I came across an article about a truck rollover accident. The truck that rolled over was filled with candy that was being dropped off at various farms for cow feed. Sugar is a fattening agent. Fatter cows produce more milk, higher sugar content milk, and larger profits.

In a recent family reunion trip to Mexico, I observed the high use of refrescos (sodas). It appeared as if there was more selection and push for it than actual water. As if that weren't bad enough, pan dulce (sweet bread) is a common breakfast item for Mexicans. Imagine the sugar intake of a refresco and pan dulce for breakfast—*enough to put you into a sugar coma.* Can you see why diabetes is prevalent in the Hispanic community? I'm saddened to learn that Mexico is high on the obese country list. Hearing that triggered a huge boost in my passion to get this message out.

GMOs and Artificially Modified Foods

Frankenfoods are "foods" that are artificial, processed, GMOs, lab-engineered, or chemical-filled (pesticides, fungicides, herbicides, hormones, antibiotics).

What are GMOs? Most of our corn, wheat, soy, many fruits, and other foods are genetically modified through laboratory processes that add a strand of new DNA, in order to modify their genetic makeup. In essence, many of our modern day flowers, plants, foods, and animals are not in their original genetic state, but have been genetically manipulated. In gardens, this can result in a very beautiful new flower or plant. However, when foods are genetically modified, it's not at all pretty.

An example of a GMO food is the product of the manipulation of a red apple to make it a purple apple, or in a natural cow creating an unnatural state of extended pregnancy, so that it can produce more milk. That may not sound like a bad thing, but if the human body is designed to run on the earth's naturally generated living fruits, vegetables, nuts, seeds, beans, and animals, then it does not have the ability to process or digest the unnaturally genetically altered products. So, how does the body process them, what does it do with them, and how does it get the nutrients it needs for optimal health?

The answer is the body doesn't know what to do with them and, in fact, is thrown into a mini jam, kind of like what happens if we insert a fake coin into a machine designed to take only quarters. Its organs can't get the nutrients they need because there are less or none in the unnatural products. The human body can't consistently, effectively, and completely push the "fake coins" through the digestive process and, as a result, can't properly eliminate (poop) them. Thus, many times the body pushes genetically altered foods to the side of an organ or intestinal lining where they stay and begin affecting the body in a negative way. Sometimes, the body even produces fibers around the item to attach it, or fat to encase it, or even attack it with our intelligent immune system, and other responses.

Eventually, this produces all kinds of results like skin conditions, fibroids, fatty deposits internally and externally, fluid retention, constipation, fatigue, allergies, weight gain, mental decline, mood depression, wear and tear on our bodies' organs and systems, and so much more. These reactions, coupled with the body's lack of receiving real nutrient-rich fuel, are a recipe for more than one health disaster. I've not even begun to discuss the nutrient depletion and health risks caused by toxins of fast food, factory-processed food, over-preserved food, sugars, caffeine, and over-the-counter and prescription drugs.

Vegetables and Fruits

Investing in natural, high integrity foods like organic (free of pesticides, added or elevated hormones, and GMOs) vegetables and fruits provides both immediate and long term benefits. Notice that I wrote "vegetables and fruits," not "fruits and vegetables." Vegetables (including herbs) provide some of the highest nutrient and fiber levels of any food.

What's wrong with fruits? Nothing is wrong with them. They are extremely hydrating, powerfully cleansing, and excellent for purifying the body and skin of toxins and blockages. As a previous sugar-addict, I have to watch my sugar intake (even natural sugar), so I limit myself to two or three fruits per day. Additionally, for those with sugar level concerns, choose lower glycemic (low sugar) fruits, such as apples, pears, grapefruit, all berries, papaya, and lemons, versus higher glycemic level fruits, such as bananas, grapes, figs, cherries, raisins, melons, and mangoes.

We get extra points for nutrient-dense and fiber-filled

cruciferous vegetables, such as *broccoli, cabbage, kale, brussel sprouts, bok choy, cauliflower, collards, radishes, turnips, watercress, rutabaga, maca, arugula, horseradish, and wasabi.* These veggies may look different, but they share remarkable similarity in that they have a very high phytochemical content. Don't let the chemical word scare you. Phytochemicals are nutrient-rich, natural earth chemicals like fiber, vitamins K, C, and E, folate, calcium, and potassium, all known to reduce risks of—and even reverse—cancer, cardiovascular disease, and other conditions.

Vegetables are best eaten in raw form; however, it would be boring to just eat salad all the time. Therefore, vegetables steamed under three minutes, sautéed with coconut oil or in grape seed oil, are wonderful too. What is also important to maximize the nutrition absorption is to have healthy fats with your veggies. Those who think opting out from salad dressing is a smart thing, I disagree. Although I would stay clear from restaurant dressings and commercial dressings as they are loaded with regular table salt, sugar, and ingredients you can't pronounce. But good ol' olive oil and vinegar are a perfect marriage with your salad.

Grains (Breads, Pastas, Cereals, and Baked Goods)

This category is probably one of the hardest things to change one's view of. Bread tastes good. It's comforting. It smells delicious when it's baking. It makes assembling food fast and varied (sandwiches, wraps, burritos, tacos, pizzas, tostadas, paninis, and breakfast treats). However, it's one of the food list's worst enemies.

One reason is, in its increasing diversity, bread has become a staple ingredient in almost every meal and creation. In addition, bread is not what it used to be. It is a hybrid of what it used to be, highly processed, and removed of vital nutrients and fiber. Gluten, a newer term in the last 10 years, is a storage protein found in wheat, barley, and rye. It is a type of food substance that can cause serious health problems in large numbers of people. But wait, isn't wheat bread better than white bread? Not necessarily. Gluten is a glue-like substance that clogs the intestines.

Many breads are now a GMO (Genetically Modified Organism), "manmade" in a laboratory where its seeds are chemically altered and "re-modified" to grow faster and bigger. Sadly, this was done without long term testing on how humans would be affected chemically, mentally, and physically. But that was not the main driver. Profits from mass production were the goal.

Carbs

Carbs have gotten a bad rap. When people say, *"I've got to cut my carbs,"* most think that means pastas, breads, and cereals. In actuality, carbohydrates are vegetables, salads, fruits, grains, cereals, coffee, colas, sweets, and sugars. So, if you "cut your carbs," you're cutting the most important foods your mind and body thrive on—vegetables, salads, and fruits. Also, if you choose sprouted, organic, whole grains in your breads and cereals, and you cut that completely out of your diet, then you're cutting a vital source of B and E vitamins, minerals, and fiber, all of which help reduce stress levels. Additionally, if someone is referring only to cutting carbohydrates from pastas, cereals, and breads, yet are still consuming cola or coffee, or sugar in their coffee, or an occasional sweet, then in reality they are consuming the most pure and direct forms of sugar and caffeine that upset blood sugar levels and the delicate hormonal balance needed for healthy mood, physical energy, mental and organ function, and sleep.

Here's the bottom line: know what carbs really are, know which of the large list of carbs you shouldn't cut, know which items harm you the most, and instead of saying, "I'm cutting carbs," say, "I'm cutting refined grains, sugars, and caffeine." When someone responds, "Oh, so you're cutting carbs," enlighten them. For some, the right "bread" can bring us life.

Proteins

We want to eat "cleaner" versions of protein, which include:

- wild-caught fish (best choices include salmon, tuna, halibut, mackerel, cod, oysters, and sardines)

- grass-fed beef, bison, and lamb

- antibiotic and hormone free, free range chicken and

turkey

- organic cage-free eggs

- plant-based protein powder-based smoothies

- organic legumes (beans, lentils, hummus, peas, peanuts)

- organic raw nuts and seeds (quinoa, chia, sesame, sunflower, flax, poppy, etc.)

- organic whole grains

- soy, but make sure that it is organic and non-GMO

Healthy Fats

Fats include nuts, seeds (sesame, sunflower, poppy, pumpkin, chia, flax, hemp, caraway, celery), avocado, coconut, and milks and oils made from them, plus cheese and fish. Not all of these are healthy for you, and not all of these that are moderately healthy should be consumed in high quantities.

Many people recognize olive oil as a good fat and end up using it to fry at high heat, which is the worst thing you can do to a good quality virgin olive oil. Olive oil is indeed a great fat that I consume daily; however, it is only for drizzling on your salad, veggies, bread, or some meats. Fry or sauté with avocado oil, coconut oil, or grape seed oil for the least levels of heat-generated rancidity or toxicity.

Be sure to check the labels on the items you buy to avoid

oils like palm, soybean, corn, and canola as their crops are heavily laden with pesticides, and the process that creates the oil is not healthy like its unprocessed whole food source. To avoid the havoc wreaked on our growing bodies and hormone function, soybeans, in particular, must be eaten in smaller quantities, in whole food form (not oil), and always organic, never GMO.

Wild-caught fish, like salmon, tuna, mackerel, and sardines are naturally rich in healthy omega fat, but not so for farm-raised. In addition, farm-raised fish are often injected with artificial dyes and other substances. They are often forced to swim in controlled and small environments, which elevate their stress chemicals, and in environments that abound in their feces. Choose wild.

Consuming dairy cheese can alter your hormone balance. It can also deposit fats in the skin and organs, resulting in weight gain, skin acne, and bad breath. Cheese made from goat milk or plant-based cheeses are good choices. If you must have dairy cheese, be sure to eat sparingly and always choose organic, non-GMO cheeses.

Real Sustainable Science

The science of food nutrition and genes is called nutrigenomics. Think of your genes as the software in your computer. They determine your body's expression of itself. Just like your computer software, your genes only do what you instruct them to do with each touch on your keyboard. Live, natural, nutrient and fiber dense food contains embedded information that talks to your genes, turning them on or off, changing their expression, and affecting their function in your mind and body, moment to moment. Imagine the messages your brain sends and receives from the input of a diet of cheeseburgers, fries, and sodas. Consider how that changes from the input of a diet of organic plant foods, wild-caught salmon, and organic sprouted quinoa.

Foods that are best for fueling our bodies are "real" foods, meaning they come from nature: from the soil (vegetables, fruits, nuts, seeds, herbs); the sky (water); the ocean (fish, ocean plants); and are organic (not altered or touched by unnatural chemicals). Pure, live, wholesome, and natural foods make us feel pure, live, wholesome, and natural. Organic produce has PLU (price look up) code labels that begin with the number series of 9. For example, #4011 is the code for a standard yellow banana. The number 9 prefix added to a PLU signifies that an item is **organic**. For example, #94011 is the code for an organic yellow banana.

Eat sustainable foods. What are sustainable foods? These are foods whose generation and harvesting use techniques that protect the environment, public health, human communities, and animal welfare. Support your local farmers. Grow your own produce. Buy in bulk (legumes, nuts, etc.), for easy storage. Choose wild-caught fish over farm-raised (that's an oxymoron; how are fish raised on a farm?). Fish need to be out in the open water, swimming freely, and eating the natural, environmentally prolific sea life, just as animals need to roam freely, grazing and eating in their organic environments.

Start your day with the most important meal of the day, breakfast! A high protein breakfast has been shown to normalize blood glucose levels and prevent bad food cravings and overeating throughout the day.

Truthfully, on occasion I do enjoy guilt-free an In-N-Out burger, an IHOP pancake, carne con chile at a Mexican restaurant, and our family's annual Christmas tamales. I know they are not considered healthy. I do this because this is part of "familia." I choose to eat them to stay connected and bond with those I love, and because I enjoy them from time to time. It's not my norm, however. I live off the 90/10 rule, or sometimes the 80/20 rule: 90% clean, 10% whatever.

Overeating

Over the centuries, despite what many people may realize, those of us in highly developed countries have been increasing the quantities of food we intake, far and above what we actually require for health and vitality. How is this possible? And why?

Many conditions underlie this state of overeating, including the stress created by the societal focus on the money, money, money; do, do, do; go, go, go; fast paced life. We wait until we're starving and then overeat. We then respond to our raised cortisol levels by eating more. We are in a hurry, so we eat fast, not realizing when we're filling up.

We're not moving our bodies and are more sedentary.

Because of this we're actually bored. When bored, we eat more. When life is harder and faster and we feel less connected, we're actually in a mildly depressed state, so we treat ourselves with food. We are more tired, so we eat to give ourselves energy.

Marketing ads teach us "bigger is better." Food establishments have lavish buffets. They tell us to say, "supersize me!" The cattle, dairy, agricultural industries, and membership chains market to consumers to buy in bulk. Container sizes and portion sizes have expanded over the generations, without our awareness, and we eat until the package is empty. It's not a conscious act. It's a slow and insidious, subliminal conditioning.

We are on far more and taking higher doses of medications than ever before in the history of mankind. Medications, along with the increasing "fake foods" we are consuming, are nutrient depleted. Thus our bodies respond to the lack of nutrients with signals for more. We misunderstand the signals asking for nutrient rich foods and fill ourselves with the same kinds of fake foods that we've become accustomed to eating.

Overeating has many origins, but the commonality is that we use food to adjust our internal chemistry, instead of making the adjustments we really need.

Absorption and Digestion

Did you know that "we are what we absorb"? How do you keep substances that you don't want to absorb out of your body? Pay attention to what you put into your mouth and what comes out the other end. It's vitally important to empty the bowel at least once a day, and completely. How do you do that? With fiber, water, exercise, sleep, and avoiding items that your body doesn't have the capacity or need to absorb.

How can you make sure you're absorbing all the nutrients in what you put into your mouth? Consider, while you may be investing in good quality vitamins, supplements, and high-quality, clean food, it is highly possible you are not absorbing it efficiently; either not eliminating it, ejecting it without being completely processed, or peeing the unused nutrients right out. What can we do to make sure our bodies absorb and digest what we eat—*even when we're eating the 10-20% items of our 90/10 or 80/20 diet?*

Here are seven steps to improve absorption of nutrients:

- Take a food enzyme right before your meals. This helps to break down your meal, so that your body can absorb the nutrients from it. In essence, we need our bodies to squeeze the nutrients into our bloodstream so they can be delivered to our entire body.

- Drink more water throughout the day, but less with your meal. What? Restaurants take your drink order first, so you can have a big pitcher of water, soda, or beer. This is actually harmful in that drinking during the meal, and within thirty minutes before and after, reduces our creation of enzymes in our tongue to absorb the food nutrients.

- Increase healthy gut bacteria (also referred as fermentation) for proper nutrition and growth. What? Isn't bacteria bad? There are bad and good bacteria. Good bacteria are essential for fighting illness, sugar addiction, weight gain, fatigue, and disease. Examples include kombucha, fermented cider, fermented vegetables, sauerkraut, kimchi, no sugar added yogurt, apple cider vinegar, jalapenos, and a high level probiotic supplement (keep your probiotic in the refrigerator to stay potent and fresh and last longer).

- Chew your food longer. Though this may not sound very appealing, chew it until you make "apple sauce," using your teeth to break down the food to absorb it faster. Yes, it's time to slow down your chow time. You will find that you will enjoy it more. It helps to put your spoon or fork down after each bite. In a hurry? Who isn't these days? Eat half of your food now and the other half later. By doing this one thing alone, you will be accomplishing two things: absorbing your food nutrients better and losing excess weight.

- Pair your foods effectively. Do you ever see someone eating a salad dry, with no dressing? They think they are doing the right thing for weight loss; however, our mindset shouldn't be on dieting, it should be on improving our health. When we eat vegetables— *cooked or raw*—our bodies absorb the nutrients better when combined with healthy fats, like olive oil, coconut oil, avocados, etc. Adding lemon and vinegar to salads and vegetables is also helpful for absorption.

- Add aloe vera to your diet. You may know aloe vera as a handy plant to have in your kitchen to handle minor burns and cuts. However, this succulent is a superfood, is great for healing the gut tissues, and can help with vitamin absorption. In a study from the UC Davis Medical Center, researchers' evaluation of the use of aloe vera showed significantly increased levels of vitamins, enhanced bioavailability, and antioxidant potential. Don't like the taste? Add a couple of spoonfuls to your morning smoothie.

- Last, but definitely not least, be happier with your life, regardless of circumstances. I can't tell you the number of people I see walking around with their heads down, their energy level down, and their thoughts down. There are things out of your control, like that person who's not nice to you or the trauma, crime, and war that we hear in the daily news. We can't change the world. But we can improve ourselves. It starts by "thinking happier." Study after study shows that looking at the bright side of things always makes us happier and healthier. Just smiling changes our physiology.

Dieting

While we're on the subjects of overeating, absorption, and digestion we need to straighten out the misunderstood concept called *dieting*. The original, true definition of "diet" is a noun, meaning (defined in various dictionaries): *the kinds of* foods and beverages that a person, animal, or community regularly consumes; *habitual nourishment; the sum of food consumed by a person or organism.*" The word "diet" is not a verb. It is not an act of doing something. It does not mean lessening the quantities of foods, or changing the types of foods one is consuming on a temporary basis to drop some pounds or inches, only to return to the way one ate before.

Diet is a lifestyle of habitual nourishment. To maintain life and a healthy, strong, self-healing, flexible feel-good body, each individual needs to listen to what their body is communicating about its needs, likes, dislikes, and the way it is affected by the individual's choices.

I have seen in recent decades so many distorted beliefs about dieting and the effects of the drastic and unhealthy "diets" that uninformed people follow—including young children taught by their parents, peers, and advertisers—that are truly harming their bodies, minds, and emotional-hormonal-chemical balance.

One of the many sad and distorted "healthy" diets promoted by so-called experts, product promoters, and food industries followed by unsuspecting, uneducated people is the trendy K diet. In my work at the Wellness Shop, we have seen so many customers come in very ill from following the K diet. This is a recommended act of eating that promotes dangerously excessive fat and animal meat and dangerously little fresh, fibrous vegetables and fruits. Initially, those who try it lose weight, but the inner organs become taxed from overworking to try to process the excessive fats, animal meats, and hormones that the human body is not designed to consume at those levels and quantities. As a result, eventually, the accumulated toxins and processes affect their gallbladder, kidney, and liver with disastrous consequences, not to mention all the weight they initially lost is gained back.

So why the diet revolution? There are many factors that create the proliferation of these and other diets that never accomplish what people are really wanting. To explain it in as few words as possible, the reason diets are so heavily recommended and followed really comes down to: *the desire for power and money, people's habits of following the crowd, a desire for a quick fix, lack of understanding about the body and true health, and a lack of true love and respect for the body and its capacity and limits.*

All of the information in this chapter is a resource guide for knowing what fuel the body needs, wants, and will thrive on for a long, healthy life, why these recommended fuels work, and why other foods and beverages do not.

Here's the bottom line: there really is no need for a diet, only a lifestyle that uses **food as medicine**. Live, organic, earth-grown, energy active foods have potent powerful enzymes, fiber, electrolytes, vitamins, hydration, elixirs, and phytochemicals that provide the body everything it needs. If there is a temporary shift when one doesn't follow the lifestyle, all that is needed is to get back on it and the body will adjust exactly as it needs.

Change Your Food, Change Your Life

One of the most powerful tools you have to change your brain and your health is what you put into your mouth. You may have heard the expression, *"we are what we think."* True positive thoughts bring positive conditions. Equally as important is, *"we are what we eat."* Food is not just calories or energy. Food is one of the fastest acting and most powerful medicines you can take to change your life. The foods you eat are the keystrokes that determine how your brain expresses its messages to your body, moving closer to health or moving toward disease.

As I was pumping gas recently, I saw a food advertisement, "Fountain Drinks $0.99! Any Size, Every Day!" Wow, that's cheaper than bottled water. Sadly, many will make that choice. Life is what you make of it. In every moment you have a choice. How do you want to feel? How do you want to look? How do you want to function? Knowing what you know now, what choices will you make?

5

Why is Sleep Underrated?

There is nothing like a good night's sleep. You know it, you feel it, you look it. Sleep is one of the fundamental components that contribute the most to your overall health. Yes, from time to time we will have less than adequate sleep. However, if you constantly deprive yourself—*whether through your own volition (uncontrolled stress, TV, social media, poor planning for a test or assignment, etc.) or through an unexpected life crisis, disease, or pain*—you are chipping away at your neurological and metabolic health, with long term consequences. Regardless of what age range you are in (child, teen, adult, senior), **sleep matters!**

The best measure you have to know if you are sleeping long enough and well enough is the condition you are in when you wake up. If you feel refreshed, relaxed, recharged, and ready to take on your day, you slept well! According to a 2013 international poll conducted by the National Sleep Foundation (NSF), less than half of those surveyed reported sleeping well every night. A lot of people have trouble sleeping.

I know firsthand about insomnia and how it can wreak havoc in your life—*and how it can make you fat.* In the past, I averaged three or four hours of nightly sleep for many years, even using over-the-counter and prescription aids, but to no avail. I'd consume about five cups of coffee the next day to stay awake. What a vicious and dangerous cycle. I attribute a large portion of the success of my health transformation to improving my sleep as it had a positive domino effect in many other areas of my health.

Benefits of sufficient and deep sleep include:

- stress reduction
- increased fat loss and muscle tone
- longer life span
- higher alertness, intelligence level, concentration, and overall mental development
- less risk of auto accidents
- less risk of heart disease, diabetes, and other heart and blood conditions
- lower appetite (doesn't promote excessive insulin secretion which leads to body fat storage)
- greater happiness (hormones)
- greater memory retention
- better, more even moods and reduction in depression

In addition to these great benefits, if you are in deep sleep through the *magical hours of 10 pm to 3 am,* you receive these additional amazing gifts:

- Healing: your body innately knows what it needs to heal, and during these hours your body is healing what's not functioning correctly.

- Anti-aging: during this rejuvenating time, your old cells are replaced with the new cells your body is producing to keep you young and healthy looking.

- Fat burning: initially, this one shocked me; I was under the impression that fat was only burned when you sweat, urinate or eliminate. Actually, during these magical sleep hours, your body is actively burning unwanted fat.

Deep sleep during the time period of 10 pm to 3 am is critical. This is not to say that we should get up at 3 am. It means those five hours for deep sleep are crucial. During the hours of 3 am to 6 am, your body is providing psychological repairs. A good night's sleep consists of six to nine hours, based on your age, level of health, and other body needs. Being asleep between 10 pm and 6 am is ideal.

Think you can sleep less during the week or pull all-nighters and make up for it during the weekend, or after the first of the month? You have been misinformed. Here's a hard fact: *you cannot make up sleep.* Your circadian rhythm (internal clock) cannot be turned back like our watches at the end of Daylight Savings Time. Sure, you can take a nap, sleep longer the next day, or sleep in on weekends, but you cannot make up lost sleep. That's not to say that a daily siesta for 20 or 45 minutes does not contribute to optimum health, but it can't replace what has been lost. Daily loss of sleep is daily loss of health benefits.

On top of that, lost sleep is cumulative. That means the hours you miss roll over and add on to the next period of lost hours. If you miss two hours a night, five nights a week, four weeks a month, twelve months a year, that adds up to 480 hours of lost sleep in just one year!

I cannot stress enough how critical this is to your health. I remember being part of an MLM (multi-level marketing) company years ago that promoted we go to bed much later every day, to work on our leads. I wish I could go back and smack that person for encouraging us to do that!

Adverse Effects of Insufficient Sleep

Sleeping less than seven hours for adults has shown an increased risk of critical disturbance to the body and brain, causing weight gain, increasing impulsive behavior, and the potential for memory loss. Increased risk of diabetes, high blood pressure, thyroid deregulation, and even premature death are also side effects of insufficient sleep.

The adverse effects of chronic sleep loss on your health is not new. Studies indicate that people who don't sleep enough are more prone to getting colds. The average adult gets two to four colds every winter (more if you have small children). Studies show that losing even small amounts of sleep per night can have surprisingly high long-term consequences on your health—*and your waistline*. Night shift workers tend to have greater risk and the onset of health concerns, due to the interruption of their circadian rhythm, the body's internal clock. They may be paid a bit more for working the night shift, but their health pays a higher price.

The Hormone Connection

Dr. Pedram Shojai, a master of meditation and natural health, shared a study from Weill Cornell Medical College showing that losing as little as 30 minutes of sleep per night on weekdays might lead to the development of obesity and Type 2 diabetes. Eating right and exercising regularly help ward off both stress and belly fat, but only if you are getting enough sleep.

Adequate sleep helps regulate good hormone patterns, thereby increasing overall feelings of well-being. Our body's hormones regulate metabolism, growth, development, tissue function, sexual function, reproduction, sleep, and mood. Skimping on sleep causes levels of the stress hormone cortisol to rise, along with levels of deep abdominal fat. There's a definite association between lack of sleep, increased stress hormones, and weight gain.

Due to the body's cortisol levels being lowest around 11 pm, going to bed by 10 pm seems to be better for ease in falling asleep. To benefit from this natural rhythm of your body's chemistry, be in bed by 10 pm and you will be asleep before the 11 pm hormonal dip. If you have trouble doing that it's because your circadian rhythm is off. This rhythm is the body's "biological clock" or "body clock." It regulates eating, sleeping, body temperature, and hormone production. Sleep deprivation disrupts our circadian rhythms, as well as too much caffeine, sleep and alert inducing prescription medications, lack of natural light, etc. Disruption of our circadian rhythms can result in mood disorders, sleep disorders, cognitive deficits, and metabolic syndrome.

Sleep loss affects your glucose tolerance, meaning your ability to handle sugar without complications. Sleep deprivation over time equates to prediabetes. On the subject of eating, our bodies produce leptin, a natural hormone that triggers our satiety (feeling of fullness). When we are sleep deprived, however, we produce less leptin. This delays our recognition of when our bodies are full. Simultaneously, our bodies produce more ghrelin, the hormone that triggers hunger. Put two and two together: not registering fullness + eating more = gaining more weight.

When sleeplessness is a problem that cannot be remedied through various efforts, it can be a sign of imbalances, such as menopause, weak thyroid, or other health conditions.

Causes of Sleep Loss

In an attempt to study sleep trouble, technology has produced gadgets that measure sleep patterns, but these gadgets emit EMFs (electromagnetic fields) which transfer low level radiation into the body and disrupt sleep, so it's a Catch-22. Many of my Wow! students used to wear smart watches until, after learning about the effects of excess EMFs, they realized the watches only add additional radiation to their already overcharged bodies. A few have opted out of them, or put EMF radiation neutralizing dot.

Overworking our central nervous systems are one of the most prevalent causes of loss of quality and sufficient sleep. It's commonly seen in the younger generations as having their mindset of indestructibility. They go to sleep after midnight and wake up at noon. Technology's 24/7 availability has not helped our health with the constant temptation to text, check social media and email, take selfies, work on or offline, and be lured into gossip, trends, news, video, and voyeurism. Information overload is overwhelming. Yes, we have to "catch up" to lessen the email inbox, news updates, and postings sometimes; however, for the sake of their health and developing brains, it's critical that our young ones get their full sleep cycle.

Natural Remedies for Better Sleep

Here are some basics that we can all do, at no cost. I'm blessed to live in Southern California, which has some of the best weather in the nation and the world.

Sunlight naturally directs our circadian rhythms. Exposure to bright light during the day activates the brain's hypothalamus and pineal gland to regulate melatonin production. For this reason, sunlight is a vital component to the body's natural ability to fall asleep, sleep deeply, and wake up refreshed.

Eat well. The better nutrition you consume, the more balanced your hormones will be, so the more relaxed your body will be for sleep. And vice versa; if you don't sleep well, your hormones become imbalanced and stop alerting you, which then causes overeating. It's a vicious circle: eating to try to sleep = chemical imbalance = sleep interference = excess hunger.

Good sleep routines are so important. Create one and stick to it. Get used to going to bed at or near the same time each evening. If you are one of those people who finds it hard to pull yourself away from what you're doing, then set an alarm to allow enough time for a before bed relaxation routine and heed it!

Stress is the silent killer and in our continually changing and quickening world, it comes from all sides. Learn stress reducing techniques. Lessen your sources of stress or it will lessen you.

Speaking of stress, the energetic stress that comes from EMF producing devices (cell phone, Wi-Fi box, computer, television, etc.) taxes your central nervous system and sleep hormones. The same applies for lights, including blue light. A Harvard study determined that any light at night negatively affects your sleep cycles, and blue light is the strongest. Eliminate all EMF devices and all lights, even tiny dots of light, laser light, and electrical appliance light from your bedroom. If you must have one in your room, seek out a blue light reduction app for your phone, laptop, and TV. You'll notice a difference in your melatonin levels and ease in falling asleep.

Mind chatter is one of the most common modern day

causes for difficulty falling or staying asleep. Nip this in the bud by writing your to-do list an hour or more before bed, to release those thoughts and free your mind and body. Then, take an honest look at that to-do list and discern which items are not really necessary, or providing value to you, or are over-giving, or are a habit of proving that you're busy enough to be respected. Where are your points of view about your to-do lists coming from? Drop them from your list. Allow more downtime for yourself. This will help center you and lessen the mind chatter.

Release and forgive the wrong and wrongdoer that crossed your path today and before. You may not consider this as a sleep remedy, but try it and see. It's kind of magical.

The following are additional natural practices to get a better night's sleep:

- Reduce caffeine and alcohol levels three to five hours before bedtime.

- Avoid eating after 7 pm.

- Exercise earlier in the day, not later at night.

- Create a quiet bedroom. Use a filter or water fountain to mask distractive neighborhood sounds and create a meditative environment.

- Drink non-caffeinated herbal tea.

- Apply lavender essential oil on your big toes, in the palm of your hands as aroma therapy, and over your pillow with a lavender/water spray or diffuser.

- Lower your bedroom temperature at night, and do this naturally (crack your window open for a breeze).

- Get outside in the sunlight every day (during "safe sun" time) for an hour or more.

- Refrain from brain stimulating technology after 8 or 9 pm (TV, computer, cell phone, video games, etc.).

- Shower or bathe (showering at night can have a reverse effect for some individuals; baths are more calming).

- Create a dark bedroom. Turn off any lights, including night lights, appliance lights, room deodorizer lights, and LED lights from your room. Get blackout shades.

- Instead of using your phone as an alarm clock, use a battery or electric clock (and use soothing music versus harsh music in your alarm choice).

- Journal before bedtime (three great things that happened to you that day).

- Read a good book / devotional (not the news).

- Pray or meditate.

- Read nightly positive affirmations to set your mind at peace.

- Do calming yoga poses or stretches.

- Drink warm milk (or dairy free milk) or golden milk

(with turmeric and honey) before bed.

- Wear pj's that are loose, instead of tight around the body, to allow for plenty of ventilation to your breast, genital, and underarm areas. (I read an article long ago that recommended the best way to sleep is completely naked, though not everyone likes that choice.)

- Sleep on your right side to activate your vagus nerve (part of your central nervous system).

Enjoy the following natural herbs and supplements to induce relaxation, sleep, and rebalance your internal rhythms:

- magnesium (relaxes muscles, soft tissue, and the central nervous system)

- lavender (calms)

- chamomile (calms and induces relaxation and sleep)

- valerian (sleep)

- passionflower (calms/relaxes)

- ashwagandha (helps anxiety, stress, etc.)

- holy basil (helps balance blood sugar and cortisol)

- melatonin (sleep)

- hops (nourishes nervous system)

Ideally, we want to go to bed around the same time each

night and wake up naturally, without an alarm clock or being awakened by anyone in the morning. Once you get into a routine, falling asleep and waking at around the same time will happen naturally. Until then, you can use an alarm clock as a backup, to be up in time for work, but try to get up naturally as soon as you can.

Just a week or two of better sleep can make a massive difference to so many different elements of your well-being and all areas of your life. So really gift yourself more sleep time. Waking up refreshed, relaxed, and early enough to start your day with plenty of time to ease into it is worth skipping the late-night TV. Turn yourself into your bed an hour earlier to reap lots of benefits. You'll love the difference!

Now you know the amazing and profound importance of sleep and the ways to get it. It's one of those things that, as you get wiser, you give more importance to (notice I didn't say "as you get older"!). The impact of sleep loss on your vitality, mood, creativity, production, inner motivation, weight, focus, body, stamina, strength, beauty, and longevity are more than ample reasons to shut down your cell phone, computer, TV, drinks, and late night conversations (including those in your mind), don't you think?

Recently, we had a guest speaker at our church, Alexis Garcia-Irons, who spoke about the importance of rest. She said, "Resting from our work is important to become *who we are*." She inspired us to reconsider what rest can do for our true identity.

One more note: when it's time for you to turn off your light to go to sleep, make sure to turn off "the light to the world" too. Don't worry; it will be waiting for you in the morning.

Rest well.

6

Why is Movement Key?

I once heard someone on the radio say the four magic words to good health are: "Eat Less and Move More." I will agree they are four important words, no doubt. However, it takes a lot more than four words to sift through all the methods, techniques, authorities, and recommendations to figure out what each of us needs to do that will really work...and that we'll actually stick to.

I personally didn't used to care for exercise, or any kind of prolonged movement for that matter. Even worse was the thought of getting all sweaty and yucky. There was one diet program I fell in love with that promised success without any exercise. How wrong was that! If anyone promises some magic pill that will make us lose weight, and get firm and tone, all without exercise of some kind, run the other way. They are straight out lying, or selling a dangerous drug or procedure that will end up costing far more than money.

Remember that thing called **movement**? Believe it or not, we were actually meant to move. And climb. And swim. And stretch. And squat. And hang. And jump. We're also meant to sweat. Cavemen didn't have cars, public transportation, bikes, or even horses to move them. They just moved. They moved their shelter, their weapons, their food sources, their bodies, and in many cases, they moved to save their lives. We're not living in caveman times, and it's been a while since any of us has been chased by hungry tigers. But, why are so many of us not moving anymore, let alone climbing, jumping, hanging, squatting, running, swimming, or walking?

Our modern technological informational age has created a double-edged sword. While we've seen unprecedented advances, we've also created a lifestyle resulting in millions of previously mobile humans reduced to sitting in a house, office, lab, warehouse, or think tank. We are the sedentary, but in a hurry, "drive-thru" generation who seems to want to touch and handle a select number of objects and tasks.

We sit holding our mobile phone because we no longer have to stand up and walk to the phone that used to sit on the table in the next room, and we lay on our sofa with an electronic device on our belly that provides all sources and methods of communication and research that we used to have to read in books, maps, or even visit a library to get. We drive through buildings designed for us to buy ready-made food fast (aka "fast food") and automated teller machines to pick up and deposit paper money from institutions who electronically handle our financial transactions.

We pick up our clothes from people who wash them for us with no water (aka "dry cleaners"; how does that work anyway?). We drive through coffee houses to purchase one of 40 varieties of caffeinated, decaffeinated, or sweetened beverages and packaged "food products" with a list of ingredients that require a magnifying glass to read and that promise to keep us awake, energized, and productive. We go through automated car wash buildings that wash our cars while we sit inside of them eating our fast food, drinking our caffeine, transmitting virtual messages, holding virtual meetings, and conducting virtual financial transactions on our mobile phones. Then, we arrive home and are too tired to wash our hair, so we apply a powdery spray that comes out of a can on our hair that promises to wash it with no water (I'm still not sure how that works).

We barely have to get out of our cars or leave our buildings. Moving is close to becoming a lost ART. Going outdoors has become a recreational activity that we plan ahead for, or call a friend to join us. It's quite possible that drive in theaters died long before their time.

I hope reading this is creating some kind of movement in you, maybe in your gut area from, you know, laughter—that ancient practice that uses abdominal muscles, releases endorphins, and happens when we are tickled by something so funny it moves us. Now, you should know that I've been sitting in this chair for hours (minus eating and bathroom breaks). Just kidding. I've actually learned to love exercise. I just had to find the right kinds, the ones that *move* me mentally and inspire me to do it. Therefore, I much prefer to use the word **movement** instead of exercise.

All joking aside, this chapter topic is something we all need to take seriously. NASA did. When they discovered that astronauts lose muscle mass after being encapsulated and out of the earth's gravity for up to two years, they knew they had to do something, and they did...vibrational machines. They actually work! (More on that later.)

The reality is not only has our modern automated lifestyle contributed to a vast decline in healthy choices, but also a steep decline in basic body movement. Our cores (the center of our bodies) are becoming dangerously weak, which affects our entire body movement, strength, and balance. We're in an age where fitness experts who specialize in breathing, posture, stretching, ergonomics, and movement are instructing us how to stretch our bodies and *move* in ways we've become incapable of or forgotten. These include proper lifting, sitting, standing, turning, squatting, lunging, bending, pulling, and other movements they call names like "Human Core Movement," "Breath for Life," or "Beginner Stretching."

Unfortunately, many people don't have the discipline to exercise. Perhaps finding the right gym may be a step in the right direction. Be careful with annual gym memberships that are bought in January. Promising to go regularly can become another expensive unchecked to-do list if we're the least bit dissatisfied or inconvenienced by the choice we've made. Gym memberships that are paid annually up front discourage us from mentally seeing the monthly deduction come out of our hard-earned money. If possible, do invest in a personal trainer to teach you how to use the machines properly and guide you through certain movements, as it is key to preventing injury.

I also love the idea of buying in home exercise equipment. We have a vibrational machine, treadmill, jump rope, circulation hand machine, free weights, etc. We just want to make sure we'll use what we buy, as an unwise purchase can soon become the best clothes hanger, before heading to the garage to collect dust and cobwebs. Then, after a few years, when our spouse nags us, we end up selling it at the next garage sale. Exercise equipment pieces are the most sold items at garage sales.

"Sitting is the next smoking." That may sound pretty extreme, but the truth of the statement is that lack of movement, especially sitting for long periods of time, is a road to disaster of all proportions. A great commitment is to get up every hour from our seated work position to stretch, go to retrieve something, jump rope, shoot some hoops, lift some weights, jump on a mini trampoline; or walk around the cubicle, halls, building, or block. Our bodies will pay us back handsomely by being more energized, flexible, and strong...and last longer!

Don't have money for expensive memberships, equipment, or groups? No matter. I recently read in *Your Amazing Itty Bitty Heal Your Body Book,* authored by my friend and colleague, Patricia Garza Pinto, a suggestion for free strength training in our own back yard. Bring home a few various sized rocks or small boulders and, with proper leg squatting and back posture, practice picking them up, carrying them across the yard, and placing them back on the ground. Repeat this as many times as possible. I have been trying it and I'm actually having fun! It is surprising how much strength, balance, and endurance can be built up using this simple, cost-free movement exercise. Remember to use the proper leg squatting and back posture to prevent injury. There are many other no cost or low cost activities you can probably find on the internet. Choose things you can have fun with or that bring some joy to you.

Core

Another great investment is a big exercise ball. Using these balls properly provides a lot of great workouts and core stabilization. A suggested goal to aim for is to be able to lift weights while kneeling on the ball without holding on to anything. You can start slow and put the ball in a cage rack, to allow yourself to hold on to something as you get stronger. Or you can practice on a carpet or grass area with nothing around that could injure you if you fall. This is not an overnight feat, but, once conquered, it brings amazing confidence in your ability and strength. Take extra caution when using these types of balls as falls are *not* recommended!

Walking is wonderful. I walk almost every morning and night after dinner. First I walk my dog, then I bring her home and take off for another round of faster paced steps. This is part of "me" time, and that cool air feels wonderful. For more intense movement/sweat, mornings are fabulous: we cool off easily, we're not tired from the end of the day, and we're not revved up by evening exercise.

Investing in a movement tracker or pedometer is a great way to keep challenging yourself and keep moving. This works well to ensure a minimum goal of 10,000 steps in a day, which is considered "active." Several Wow! students suggested using a cell phone app to count steps, but that's not my recommendation as it means your cell phone has to be on your body all day long (too much radiation—more on that later). Other great fitness investments include an inversion table, sauna, AVACEN (advanced vascular circulation enhancement machine), etc.

Here's a fun piece: a mini trampoline. Nicely priced starting around $50, they are a great bang for our buck. Not only do they get us moving, oxygenated, circulated, energized, and thinking clearly, but they also get us feeling happier in a few minutes. And the best news is they are just about the number one way to get our lymphatic system moving and clearing toxins in our bodies. When our lymphatic system moves and clears, our skin clears, our digestive system moves and eliminates, our body recharges, and we feel lighter.

If you want to take it to the next level of cell movement— hence the important circulation we need—try a **vibrational plate**. Using this plate highly reduces the possibility of a fall compared to the trampoline and even helps to unwind as all you do is stand on it and you get "jiggled out." Our health improves exponentially with the daily use of these types of equipment. I can't recommend these little powerhouses highly enough.

Whatever our style, we need to choose the type of movement or exercise that will motivate us. I get bored easily, so I need to be changing my routine, group class, method, etc.

As for sweating? Sweating is a necessary part of staying fit, healthy, and detoxed, so I "got over it," as my husband told me many times, suggesting I learn to love sweat.

Stretching

What does movement have to do with posture? Lack of movement, strengthening exercises, and stretching shrinks our muscles, hunches our backs, pushes our heads forward, compresses the discs between the vertebrae in our spine, and tightens our ligaments and tissue. What does all this lead to? Shrinkage!

Our bodies are like cars. If a car has been hit in an accident, side swiped one too many curbs, or landed with a jolt off a high hill or other impediment, we take it to get an alignment. What happens if we don't? In time, we start hearing noises, tires start wearing unevenly and more quickly, metal pieces start clicking, and in severe cases the car's appearance is noticeably off. We've all seen it; a truck or car is driving down a straight highway in front of us, but it looks like it's going slightly sideways. If we treat our bodies like that, without getting realigned by a chiropractor after we've had an injury, fall, or car accident, we're asking for trouble.

On the subject of shrinkage, women shrink more than men, an average of two inches after 40 years, while men shrink an inch and a half. Here are some ways we can minimize this:

- stretch every day
- pay attention to posture
- eat healthfully
- see a chiropractor regularly
- stay hydrated

Poor posture ages us. Most older people start showing signs of posture decline in the hunch of their upper back and the forward tilt of their head. Don't be one of them. Roll your arms back, push up your chest, and feel an imaginary cord pulling the top of your head toward the sky.

Other Holistic Modalities (Chiropractor/Massage/Acupuncture)

Our whole family loves chiropractors, although I grew up with a negative notion about them. They all have different hands and techniques, so find what feels best to you and your wellness needs. I am very glad through education and trying different hands that we now have amazing experiences with chiropractors and this holistic approach is definitely part of our "wellness path." The same goes with professional massages. Not only do they feel good, but they are incredibly good for your lymphatic system. A word of caution: if you are trying a professional massage for the first time, start slow as you might be very sore the next day while your body adjusts to these approaches.

Acupuncture originated in ancient China and involves pricking the skin or tissues with needles. It's used to alleviate pain and to treat various physical, mental, and emotional conditions. Acupuncture is an excellent approach as well.

Travel

Comfortable shoes are a must to walk well between flights, in your hotel, or final destination. Bands are an easy way to have something to do movements. Or the quick thing: find an online video with your favorite movement, or at least a 5 to 10-minute breathing meditation. Hint: our bodies know when we travel and often hold back from having a bowel movement so pack some cascara sagrada herb capsules for relief.

Digestion

Digestion, digestion, digestion, is just as important to health as location, location, location is to real estate. I specifically put this topic under the "movement" chapter because digestion is literally the *movement of stuff* on the inside, with a goal to *move it* out. I cannot overstate how important this is to our overall health. Think about this. We eat an average of three meals per day, not to mention snacks. Logically, it makes sense that we would eliminate/discard the waste three times a day, right? Here lies the problem. Many eliminate on average one time every two days. Yuck!

How uncomfortable that must be! The average American has 25 pounds of elimination stuck in their colons. The autopsy of the beloved actor, John Wayne, revealed 40 pounds of waste stuck in his intestines! The bottom line is if we are not eliminating at least one to two times daily, we are full of crap!

Our gut is considered our second brain. Rightly so. It has such an important job to do with all the fuel we put in our mouth daily and then squeeze through 22 feet of small intestine so we can **absorb** the nutrients of the food, then another six feet in the large intestine to prepare for final elimination. That's a lot of work. Something just as important to know is that our emotions are primarily housed in our gut and as the famous stress rollercoaster goes up and down, so does our digestion patterns. Sadly, even if we are eating all organic foods, if we don't control our stress levels, then it can negatively affect our digestion system; hence, not getting rid of our waste on a daily basis which leaves that waste to putrefy (screaming toxins).

What Can Aid Digestion?

- Apple cider vinegar (never take straight; 1-2 teaspoons in diluted in 4-6 ounces of water).

- Drink more water (room temperature is best for digestion).

- Eat more fibrous foods (leafy greens and other veggies, both raw and cooked, and fruits like apples).

- Move, move, move…exercise helps the colon get going.

- Take psyllium husk or other fiber.

- Cut back on constipating foods (meats, cheeses, breads, sweets, etc.).

- Jump on a trampoline daily.

- Eat slower and use your non-dominant hand (trust me, it works).

- Don't drink fluids with meals (more on this below).

- Take sips of water and swish it around in the mouth to activate hydrochloric acid.

- Herbs like cascara sagrada, licorice root, and magnesium.

- Ivy's Famous Colon Cleanse (ivys.com)

Regarding my recommendation not to drink fluids with meals, most of us would say, "What? That's ridiculous. How are we supposed to eat and get our food down?" That's the point. If we can't get the food down through the process of our natural chewing, the saliva that our mouths naturally create, the choice of foods we eat, not waiting till we're starving, and slowing down, then we are doing it wrong.

I know, the first sentence out of the mouth of our server when we go out to eat is, "What would you like to drink?" What most of us are not taught is that our tongue and mouth creates saliva through the process of chewing, which contains digestive enzymes designed to break down our food efficiently for swallowing and digesting. When we drink fluids with our meals (or immediately before or after our meals), our digestive enzyme process stops. But wait...

I have to hand it to my dad. We all thought it was strange because he never drank any liquids when he was eating. You were right on this one, Dad! He had another good habit that I wondered about. He always rinsed his mouth out after a meal. I used to think that was strange too, but that habit is actually responsible for preserving his full set of teeth up to his passing. Okay, two health points for you, Dad!

One area of movement we can slow down is eating. Slow down! This is very important in helping with digestion as our mouths will have time to create the salivary enzymes so important in digestion. We will also have a fuller sensation as we go to actually "taste our food" versus swallowing it quickly.

One last note on the benefit of exercise, digestive movement, and movement of any kind: we will definitely get a better night's sleep. The key to remember is to Move Our Bodies!

7

What Toxins?

Simply put, a toxin is a poisonous substance. We can get them from the food we ingest, the water we drink, the air we breathe, the chemical products we use in our jobs and chores, our homes, and even our emotions. This list goes on and on. For example, if your appendix bursts, toxins are released into your blood stream, but excess emotional and mental stress can also increase toxic chemicals into the body. Yet, this human body we've each been given is designed to handle a certain amount of toxicity. Health problems start to occur in the case of toxic overload, poor nutritional status, and the individual's ability or inability to excrete the toxic elements. It is important to remember that it's impossible to remove every harmful chemical from the body and there is no perfectly "clean" place on Earth to live. Hence the goal is to find balance in our overall well-being, our Wellness Path.

My definition of DISEASE is an accumulation of TOXINS.

I've broken it down to the three major toxin groups:

Food and Water: an overload of "manufactured" food (aka frankenfoods) which is so far away from REAL LIVE (clean) food that comes from soil to provide energy and life.

Manufactured food is considered food from boxes, containers, and bags. In other words, prepackaged food which contains many chemicals to enhance flavors (making it addicting), appearance (food color), and added preservatives so they have a long shelf life and to not lose money by products expiring soon. Also, too much caffeine, sugar, breads, dairy, etc.

Instead of drinking water from tap or plastic bottles, consider better water that has a good pH level with no fluoride, chlorine, etc. Even the water you shower in can be very toxic to your skin and hair. For a small investment, you can add a shower filter.

Where do you start? Begin by making wiser food and beverage choices that come **closer to Nature**. Your investment in organic foods and good quality water will improve your health in the long run.

Environmental: Carpeting, plastics, pollution from cars, laundry ingredients, smoking, EMFs (radiation), artificial fragrance gadgets like sprays, plugins, candles; beauty products, cleaning supplies, prescription drugs, toiletries, Teflon pans, poor air quality due to indoor pets (sorry!), etc.

Note: it was once calculated that a woman leaves her home with an "average of 500+ toxins" every morning!

Where do you start? On your skin, use shampoo, soap, etc., that are paraben-free (no preservatives) and deodorant with no aluminum. Avoid sleeping with your cell phone, remove computers from your bedroom, have live plants and salt lamps near TVs and computers, use essential oils (my favorite brand is Young Living) to improve energy, buy room fragrance and household cleaners free of chemicals, and place EMF radiation dots on your cell to help neutralize radiation.

Mental/Emotional: This includes always being stressed, negative thoughts, constantly feeling overwhelmed, adrenal overload, toxic relationships, and too much running around yet feeling unproductive.

From a spiritual standpoint this would be lacking purpose and meaning, too many and too long "to do" lists," not saying "no" enough, not releasing past emotional trauma, etc.

Past blunt force traumas from car accidents, surgeries, vaccines, tattoos, piercings, and other traumas directly to the physical body can leave lasting damage. Dr. Bob Marshall called this damage, "interference fields," which prevent the body from absorbing nutrition in that area so it doesn't heal fast or at all in some cases. Even worse, the interference fields can diminish or turn off the functioning of major organs.

Where do you start? Use herbal and natural brain supplements such as ashwagandha and chamomile, incorporate daily "movement," get better sleep, practice positive affirmations, go in for chiropractic adjustments, use Young Living essential oils for balance, make up your mind to let go of little things, FORGIVE and move on, and hang around with positive thinking and healthy people. I know it sounds easy, but toxic people, including those special relatives, can easily hinder your health. If you have no choice and have to live with them, make up your mind to set the appropriate boundaries.

Seek help from experts that can teach you new habits to overcome ongoing or recurring concerns. If your car sounds like it's going to break down, you hurry to an expert, the mechanic, to repair it so you can move on with your life. How different is that from our health? Let's not wait till we hear the diagnosis or see the red lights of the ambulance. Let's love ourselves enough to seek help or solutions. The Wow! Program is known for its great love, laughter, and uplifting energy to help along the healing journey.

Removal and Prevention

Removal of toxins is possible through flushing the body, internal use of products to diffuse and expel toxins, external application of such products, and shifting emotions into a positive state. Determining which one(s) to use depends on what the source of the toxin is.

While there are many ways to remove toxins, one of my favorite ways is using the famous "Ivy's Cleanse," which is a gentle and effective way to eliminate some of this bad stuff. After all, isn't this what bowel movements are meant to do—rid our waste? Some of the natural ingredients include aloe vera, chlorophyll, psyllium hulls, etc. The important part is in the combination and frequency of the cleanse. Drinking plenty of good quality water is also key to help flush it out too. Be careful; I have also seen other very harsh one-time cleanses that leave you stuck on the toilet all day—that's no fun, or productive.

Additionally, you can remove many toxins through the use of saunas which sweat it out. We just talked about exercise (movement) in the last chapter.

More importantly, how do we prevent them?

The obvious answer is by **reducing toxin intake**. It may be simply said but not necessarily simply done. It requires a mind shift of wanting to make not one change but several, more like a "transformed lifestyle."

Some examples include:

- plastic shower curtains replaced with cloth ones or BPA-free material plastic
- different color, round plastic bath sponges that hang on a string replaced with a loofa (plant) sponge
- outlet fresheners or aerosol spray fresheners replaced with essential oil diffusers
- common, small daily blood thinner pill (apple cider vinegar can do wonders)

Preventing or Reversing Emotional and Mental Stress and Their Toxins

One way to reduce toxins is to reduce stress. Here are a

few options:

- Deep breathing is one of the easiest ways.

- Green tea has been proven to boost health in many ways, from fighting cardiovascular disease and obesity, to preventing Type 2 diabetes and even some forms of cancer. An added bonus: it makes you feel good! Green tea contains L-theanine, an amino acid that naturally lowers blood pressure and anxiety levels. Due to caffeine levels, it is best to enjoy before noon.

- Movement is part of any health improvement regimen and one of the fastest ways to regain lost energy. Studies show that people who exercise at least 2-3 times per week experience significantly less depression, anger, and stress than those who exercise less frequently or who never exercise.

- Music (especially vibrational music) is known to relax the mind, also known as sound therapy.

- Lavender is helpful in promoting sleep, treating mild burns, relieving pain, and calming you with a natural antidepressant that stabilizes your mood. I have personally witnessed the power of lavender. I broke my right wrist a couple years ago. Rather than filling the prescription for inflammation and pain, I treated those symptoms with my Young Living essential oils.

- Laughter really is the best medicine. Not only does a

good belly laugh loosen your muscles for a long time afterward, but it also causes the release of endorphins, feel-good chemicals that reduce stress and can even temporarily relieve pain. One study found that people who have a good sense of humor actually live longer!

Preventing or Reversing Nutritional and Chemical Stress and Their Toxins

Nutritional, stress-producing toxins come from taking in foods, drinks, drugs, medications, and other substances through eating, inhaling, injecting, or applying to the skin. Nutritional stress is also chemical stress, due to the chemical reaction of the body. Take soda, for example. It takes 35 glasses of alkaline water to neutralize the harmful chemical effects of just one soda!

What about meat or dairy foods? An overabundance of either of these in the diet changes the chemistry of our body; thereby producing stress to our cells, tissue, circulation, skin, and vital organ function. That's not even taking into account the artificial hormones, genetically produced feed, and stress producing environments and practices used in raising and slaughtering our animals for food—or the artificial preservatives, dyes, and other fillers added to the meat in the packaging process.

Western medicine is not winning the war on cholesterol. In my research, I could find no evidence that cholesterol drugs prevent heart attacks. Yet, millions are prescribed cholesterol medications. Cholesterol is naturally produced by our bodies. Our cell walls are made of it. Our brain is made of it. Vital hormones, like testosterone and progesterone, are made from it. Our bodies can't digest fat without it. Nor can our bodies produce vitamin D without it. Instead of taking drugs to "manage" out of balance cholesterol levels, I've been using real foods, especially ACV (apple cider vinegar).

Products that we use in our homes, offices, warehouses, and work environments, on our bodies, in our gardens, and in our cars contain toxins that stress the body's delicate chemical balance. Even products touted as symptom-relievers, such as stomach antacids, are stressful to the body's natural systems and healing abilities. The list of nutritional and chemical toxins and their stressful effects on the body are too numerous to list.

Here are a few of the many conditions associated with stress-producing toxins from nutritional and chemical sources:

- allergies (when allergies are prevalent, your immune system is on overload; therefore, it's imperative to build on your immune system to strengthen it)

- auto-immune disorders

- cancer

- diabetes

- high blood pressure

- heart disease

- Alzheimer's

- neuropsychiatric disorders including ADD, ADHD, anxiety, and depression

- thyroid disorders

A few tips to reduce, eliminate, or prevent nutritional and chemical toxins include:

- Avoid Teflon kitchen or other products; consider stainless steel or titanium (I love my Salad Master!).

- Use, wash, and reuse glass bottles versus plastic (this helps in two ways: prevents plastic chemicals from going into your body, and prevents BPAs from going into our environment and plastic from filling our landfills).

- Whole food dietary supplements (including iodine for the thyroid), minerals (calcium, magnesium, selenium, zinc, liquid trace minerals), and detoxifiers. My foundation includes a good multi-vitamin (no iron, unless your blood tests have proven you are anemic), vitamin C, omega fish oil, and vitamin D3.

Oral Health

Something that may surprise you is that our mouths are a breeding ground for toxins that enter our bloodstream and major organs. Healthy oral care is necessary in creating and maintaining good hygiene, skin, body scent, and beauty. Good oral health is also, and more importantly, vital in preventing illness and disease. Infections (toxins) from lack of oral care and bad diets begin in the mouth, enter the gums and the blood stream, and are transferred through the arteries that go directly to the heart. Many people don't know that one of the major causes of heart disease (and heart attacks) can be traced back to poor oral care. Sometimes this can take years and go undetected.

Here are just a few ways to prevent toxins and maintain your body chemistry and health through effective oral care:

- Floss after every meal, if possible (ask your dentist to show you the proper way to floss, to not damage the gums or miss pockets where food is trapped along the sides of the teeth).

- Softer toothbrushes are easier on your teeth and gums.

- Use fluoride-free toothpaste.

- Use sweetener-free toothpaste (no saccharin, or sugar substitutes).

- Brush immediately after consuming sugary foods or beverages.

- Avoid going to bed without brushing your teeth. Eight hours, or more, of dirty teeth will eventually and cumulatively have a serious effect on the health of the gums and teeth, and internal chemistry and organ health.

- Stay away from hard candies, caramel/taffy candies, sticky candies, sodas, and sugary juices.

- Combine aluminum-free baking soda and some drops from a lemon; let it fizz, then gently brush your teeth and rinse. Don't let this substance sit unrinsed for longer than 90 seconds. In addition to a healthy toothpaste alternative, this is also a natural teeth whitener.

- Brush your tongue, or use a tongue scraper, as well as the roof of your mouth.

- Immediately after a meal or beverage, do a quick swish with water and swallow.

Preventing or Reversing Environmental Frequency Stress and Its Toxins

Just about every household in industrialized nations has a microwave. Many years ago, a good friend's grandmother told me that microwaves caused cancer. I didn't give much thought to that, looking instead to the fact that just about every home has one, and so I brushed off her belief as an old wives' tale. How I wish that I knew back then what I know now. Microwaves do, in fact, emit radiation, which is known to cause cancer. While I have not been able to successfully get rid of mine—because it's built into the wall—and my family is not convinced enough in the research, I minimize its use.

Here are three important tips to remember if you do use a microwave:

- Don't stand within the bandwidth of its emission while it's on.

- Do not open it while it still has time remaining on the clock. Clear the time, wait a few seconds, and then open the door.

- Do NOT use any kind of plastic containers or plastic wrap in the microwave. Using plastic in the microwave actually infiltrates your body and mind with two kinds of toxins: EMFs and chemical (plastic, when heated, is highly toxic and goes directly into the food or beverage it covered and then right into your body). Wax paper or a napkin is a better choice.

In addition to a microwave, most of us own a cell phone, a laptop, tablet, or desktop computer, and an air conditioner—*or all the above.* Each of these contain and transmit electromagnetic fields (EMFs) constantly into the atmosphere. Many items like televisions, cell phones, and computers have the option of being put in "sleep mode," but they are still on and transmitting EMF waves, even when not in use. More importantly, they continue to do so even when they are turned off.

We have Wi-Fi in our homes, our workspaces, our schools

and institutions, and every retail business we walk into. We are encased in an EMF bubble in our newer cars with Wi-Fi! The increasing number of these devices in our environment only strengthens and worsens the effect these EMFs have on our health. This is something we need to pay attention to, as it will only increase as technology expands. There is a price to pay, and we have no place to hide from these EMFs.

At best, get out in nature every day, away from all electrical, electronic, and internet sources. Take extended nature trips. Go barefoot in nature. Go near or in the ocean or lakes as often as possible. Use EMF mats and body protection devices wherever possible. At minimum, leave your cell phone off as much as possible. Stand in another room when the microwave is on (better still not to use it at all).

Turn your phone off at night and put it in a room other than the room you're sleeping in. Go back to the old fashioned battery-operated alarm clock. Do not put the modem or router in your bedroom. Remove computers, televisions, and Wi-Fi devices from your bedroom. Bedrooms are meant for only two things: R&R (rest and romance). Anything else will interfere with your brain and body system's natural ability to fully disconnect, rest, deep sleep, repair, and recalibrate.

If you can't always get outside and away in nature, go out in your garden and get in the earth and dig and walk for a while, to neutralize the EMF energy in your brain and body. If you don't have a garden, live plants are very helpful in absorbing toxins in the air. Put them in all of your living, working, and playing environments—the more the better! Among the best are spider (NASA study), pothos, and ZZ plants. With the exception of the spider plant, the darker green the better—like vegetables in your diet.

Natural salt crystal has been credited with a range of curative powers, from air purification to migraine relief and defense against airborne germs. Mined in the foothills of the Himalayas where they have absorbed mineral elements that enrich them and imbue them with different colors, Himalayan salt crystal lamps and rocks release healing negative ions into the air when turned on. Similar to the energizing negative ions released in the natural settings of mountains, waterfalls, or beaches, they increase oxygen flow to the brain, harmonize and purify the room and atmosphere, help to alleviate depression, relieve stress, heal the effects of mental stress, and boost daytime energy.

These ions also naturally counteract the effects of the electromagnetic waves we are bombarded with from the devices and appliances I listed above. Salt crystal lamps have also been proven to protect against airborne germs and reduce the symptoms of allergies, sinus problems, "brain fog," and insomnia.

When I heard the term "negative ions," I thought: *Is that reversed? Shouldn't it be positive* (good) *ions?* Nope. In this case, the good ions are "negative" ions.

Here's a great book on the subject: *Himalayan Salt Crystal Lamps* by Clemence Lefevre.

Preventing or Reversing Attention Stress and Its Toxins

Are you a distraction addict? Continual mental distraction, multitasking, information overload, and technology addiction is a stress-producing toxin for the mind and emotions, as well as for the environment—a triple whammy! We might think of addictions only as alcohol, drugs, food, gambling, smoking, porn, control, etc. Isn't addiction a "compulsion," or being "hooked" on something that is "hard to let go," that you "can't do without," that "interferes with everyday life," and maybe prevents you from maintaining balance, peace, joy, and well-being? Don't these descriptions apply to our fixation, focus, and constant need to "be informed," "be productive," "be social," and "be included" through multitasking, using technology and social media, and paying attention to everything and everyone around us, as often as possible? Doesn't the continuation of this create an inability to concentrate, stay centered, be peaceful, sleep well, and stay focused on our personal well-being, and stay healthy and free of illness and disorders?

The effects of distraction addiction are prolific. Lack of deep and sufficient sleep, plus being overwhelmed from information and observation overload, keeps the brain on overload, the body in "go mode" or "download mode," and the mind on "multi-focus mode," which results in energy loss, weakness, immune stress, anxiety or mood swings, illness, and eventually, disease.

Our smart phones have us conditioned like Pavlov's dogs

(this was a famous experiment that showed dogs could be trained to salivate at a signal that was associated with being fed). We have more technology and less vitality. While I'm not willing to give up my cell phone, there are some boundaries that I've needed to set to prevent the consumption of my productivity, creativity, work, rest, health, and relationships. Here are some suggested boundaries; some may seem crazy, but ask anyone with sleeping issues how awful it feels to be chronically sleep or R&R deprived:

- Discipline yourself to shut down from all distraction at 9 pm. Allow your brain to unwind and prepare for deep sleep.

- Remove electronics from your bedroom. Your bedroom is your sacred space for sleep, rest, and romance.

- Commit to limit email reading to 2-3 times a day, with the last time being two hours before bed.

- Turn off your phone, apps, computer emails, and social media pages and groups. The relief you will feel from no longer hearing that beep or sound each time a message, story, or video is sent or posted will enable you to stay in your zone, on track for what's important to you, and enhance your life.

I'm blessed to have a small community park in our neighborhood to walk in. More often than not, I see parents spending more time on their cell phones than being present physically, mentally, and emotionally with their children. I'm always sad when I see a mom or dad pushing their child on the swings, while obsessively checking their phone the entire time. I may have done the same with my boys, but I'm grateful to have this awareness now. It's never too late, but the sooner the better. True family time doesn't include cell phone time, unless you're geographically apart and that is the only way to communicate.

One of the hardest parts of dealing with internet addiction is that, unlike booze, drugs, porn, or gambling, it's socially acceptable—*and even encouraged.* In fact, it seems as if almost every day a new technology is introduced that promises to make us "more connected." We can now check our email, social media, phone messages, and the web at any time, from any place— even our watches and our cars. How ironic. The effect of these technologies has been less connection, not more. Instead of simply being present in each moment and feeling connected with ourselves, our creativity, our imagination, our work, and our loved ones, our attention is spread across the world. I wonder what long term effect this modern lifestyle will have on family units?

I left this for last, but it is definitely not least. Natural, plant-based, medicinal essential oils, and the various methods and applications with them, have been used throughout the ages. Some oils (my favorite line is Young Living) have the ability to relax, stimulate, and create balance between the body and mind. Aromatherapy is one of the oldest non-invasive health practices. Scents have a powerful effect on the mind and body. The oil's aroma is picked up by the olfactory nerve, in the back of our nose, and sent to the brain where it affects the senses. Essential oils can evoke memories, stimulate feelings, arouse sensations, and trigger the body's natural healing processes. Due to their direct impact on the limbic system, which processes our memories, emotions, and feelings, they can also stimulate emotional responses.

Essential oils can be applied externally, added to water or food for internal use (only high food grade quality oils), diffused into a room, and used for wounds, pet needs, and hidden toxins. Due to the effects and uses of these earthy elements, they are an all-around healing and preventative resource for all types of stress. Do your research in an essential oil handbook and start receiving the benefits of their amazing healing power.

8

What's in Your Palace?

For all its convenience, advancement, and variety, life in today's Western world does not guarantee happiness, health, or fulfillment. No matter how high your limit is, Mastercard can't pay for it! Our frantic daily existence often leaves too little time to relate to one another, let alone experience the benefits of the natural world. We may even be too distracted to listen to the needs of our own bodies and struggle with rising stress levels and chronic illness, as a result. In this state, we cannot thrive. However, when we recognize the problem, and as we begin to search for integrating connection, the wisdom of previous generations can help us.

In the last few years of my deepening holistic lifestyle, I've come to realize the importance of our *palace,* more commonly referred to as our "home, house, sanctuary, casa," or "digs." I prefer the more grandeur status that *palace* implies. Our palace is a foundational component in the restoration of our health and happiness. For those who work long hours or travel a lot, it may not be the place you spend most of your time, but it probably occupies a highly valued space in your heart. I'm thrilled when I get texts and praises from my Wow! Program students about how they've learned to appreciate the importance of their home, and now refer to it as their *palace.*

Create Your Palace

Visualize yourself arriving home and entering your special space. You are the king or queen walking into your personally designed palace. To make it truly special—a palace that excites you, comforts you, protects you, inspires you, and nourishes you—it must ignite your senses.

As you step around the corner, see your clean walkway, personalized landscaping, stepping stones, planted flowers, lights, and decorations. As you enter the front door, see the beauty of your colorful walls, the sunlight on the floor, your green leafy plants, the mirror's reflection, your comfortable furnishings, and the treasured keepsakes you display.

Hear yourself say, *"Home sweet home"* as you see your children playing and your pets welcoming you. Hear the wind chimes ring in the breeze, the water trickling in the fountain, your favorite music playing, and the clock chime. Hear the peacefulness. Hear the stillness. Hear the voices of your loved ones, or the quiet of your private domain. Hear the cat's meow, the birds chirping, or the ballgame on television.

As you walk into the kitchen, taste a piece of fruit, chilled water, your favorite beverage, or—if dinner is being prepared—a bite of what's to come. Have an ample supply of your favorite fruits, vegetables, beverages, and healing snacks stocked in the pantry, refrigerator, and on the countertop. Make it more available on a tray on the dining room table, on a shelf in the living room, or even the bedroom to taste at your whim.

Smell the fresh ingredients being prepared in your meal, the dessert baking in the oven, and the woodsy, floral scent of natural candles. Smell the rich lotion you put on your hands after you've washed the stress away and the earthy fragrance of the diffuser as it sends puffs of healing essential oils into the air to clear your space, shift your energy, and envelope your senses.

Feel the touch of your pet's paw on your arm, your partner's embrace, or your child's hug wrapped around your back. Or, enjoy the softness of your pillow, throw, favorite chair, or plush rug as you spread out on it and exhale. Feel the breeze flowing in through your open window and the smoothness of your bed as you rest for a few minutes to shut off the world.

How would you create your palace, designed just for you, to refresh you, inspire, comfort, heal, and please you?

If you're rolling your eyes and thinking, *Yeah right, that's sure not my house!* then perhaps your situation is more like screaming conversations, plain gray walls, and floors covered with spilled drinks, clothes, or toys; requests to put out the trash, stacks of dishes, fake dust covered plants, flies swarming the rotted fruit, or a stinky bathroom. Don't blame the state of your palace on someone or something else.

Figure out what you want, dive in, and start making the changes. Let others know what it feels like to have a palace that soothes and nourishes all of you and what their part will be in creating and maintaining it. They will sense your energy and attitude change, and you'll be surprised at how your family or housemate will shift when they know you are serious in caring about your palace and how you all can enjoy the feel of it. *Change doesn't begin with someone else or something outside of you. It begins with YOU.*

Feng Shui Your Palace

What can we do to create our sanctuary, our palace? Here are some principles of *feng shui* (pronounced fung shway), also known as space clearing, energy lifting, or room staging. *Feng shui* is an energetic environmental science developed over 3,000 years ago in China that creates harmony in your space, turning a home, office, or any space into a tranquil sanctuary of peace and beauty that restores your spirit.

Clear the clutter. Get rid of things you don't LOVE, you don't need, you have duplicates of, are broken or damaged, have sat unused for a year or more; or don't fit you, your family, or your style anymore. Have a garage sale, pay it forward (donate), or—if the item is unusable—THROW IT OUT! Don't put this step off, as clearing is the most important step. Clutter is the number one reason for sad, scary, angry, depressing, sickening, or exhausting spaces. Clutter represents stagnant energy, a belief in "not enough," and insecurity about the future. Clutter is a state of mind, beginning and ending in the mind.

So what constitutes clutter? Anything we do not use or wear, or are keeping in case it might be needed in the future "someday" is clutter. Inherited objects and gifts given to us that we don't like but feel guilty about parting with are clutter. Anything we collect, or accept from others but don't need, or hold onto in a drawer for sentimental value, or have duplicates of and don't use, or things we didn't have when we grew up and wanted are all clutter. Artificial dust magnet fake trees, plants, and flowers, and dusty trinkets and collectible objects are clutter. This may not be something easy to give up, so take it as far as you can, one step at a time. Have someone help you.

When we hold onto objects, structures, clothing, tools, or other possessions that are falling apart, not working, in disrepair, or broken, we are asking for the negative energy to stay with us. We are accepting a life that isn't working. And we'll continue to experience things not working, whether it's a tool, a toy, a garden hose, or a living room door. It's our belief that we can't have, or may never be able to have, a life in wonderful condition. So, either repair it or replace it. If it's been sitting for a year waiting to be used or fixed, fix it or toss it. That may sound harsh, but that might be just what you need to hear to move forward.

If we are wanting something new in our lives, something different, then we need to make room for it and prepare to receive it by creating space for it. As soon as we rid ourselves of clutter that has taken up space and is not serving us, we instantly feel a sense of lightness, an opening in our world, an expansion of our breathing, an increase in our energy, and a heightened spirit of positivity and freedom. Many times, we experience some type of change in our lives, like something or someone new coming in, something that we have been wanting, or something that makes our lives happier and easier.

Beautify, Fortify, and Signify Your Palace

Does your palace have curb appeal? What does it look like when you drive up to it? Does your palace have a visible address number? Having numbers displayed on the house are not only helpful for new guests to find you, but also so that emergency vehicles aren't delayed from being able to identify your palace. Every second counts. We need to make sure our palace looks and feels like a palace, not an uncared for, uncomfortable shack. Surround your palace with only things that are functional, cared for, meaningful, beautiful, and bring you joy. It does not take a lot of money to make it clean, clear, and simple.

Enjoy good quality air. Use live, air-purifying plants, like pothos, ZZ, peace lily, and ocean spider plants—the darker green in color the better (see more of this in Chapter 7). Use an air purifier. Open your windows and feel the clearing and cleaning that occurs from the movement of the air that you breathe. This is so important if you have carpeting or pets, or if you cook a lot.

A front screen door is a must for me to keep my palace free of insects, uninvited critters, dirt, leaves, and other environmental elements. Yes, many homes are adorned with beautiful closed doors, but when we look at the health value of air flowing in and circulating through our palace, we see how valuable a screen door truly is.

Light is energizing. Light is uplifting. Use as much natural light as possible. Open the blinds, shutters, drapes, and doors, and let that light come in and naturally invigorate the space of your palace. For an extra glow in late afternoon, early morning, or nighttime, enjoy the harmony, healing, and purification of Himalayan salt lamps.

Wall pictures and art should speak to our soul about beautiful memories, love, excitement, reflection, and appreciation of life.

Colors make our palace come to life. Color choices create specific moods and feelings. Color has the ability to shift us. Be brave and choose colors that reflect your desires and your desired look. Remember that dark colors, and specific colors like red, brown, dark green, and dark gray make a space feel and look smaller, more closed in, and heavy.

Mirrors are among the least expensive decorative accessories and can make a profound difference in a room. Make a bold statement using mirrors as large gorgeous accent pieces. With so many sizes, shapes, colors, and types, choose what makes you feel good...or design your own! Mirrors combine function, art, dimension, and space enhancement, and they reflect light. Perhaps most importantly, they reflect the image that we have of ourselves, and continue to change that reflection as we shift our health and happiness. Make sure you smile when you see yourself. This simple gesture improves your well-being.

Be especially mindful and honor loving energy in three important rooms: your bedroom, your bathroom, and your kitchen, and any room you spend time in bonding, breaking bread, and having meaningful conversations. This might be your living room, family room, dining room, or patio. One of my favorite places in my palace is our 25-foot long sun room. We eat and live in that room more than anywhere else and love its fresh air surrounded by the beauty of our fruit trees, lots of grass, sun decorations, water fountain, and plenty of beautiful singing birds cruising through.

Other Palace Spaces

Do your palace possessions have names? If a possession is meaningful or helpful to you, why not name it? My car is "Latte" (she's light brown and sweet looking). My vibration exercise plate is "Jiggi" (she jiggles me a lot). My treadmill is "Nordy" (NordicTrack made her). My Vitamix blender that we use multiple times a day is "Lil' Hummer" (he's strong and bold-looking and crunches everything fast, like a Hummer running over an aluminum can).

Garages are intentionally designed to be either an area for parking or storing motor vehicles, or a commercial establishment for repairing and servicing motor vehicles. Somehow, somewhere along the way through the ages, garages have transitioned to being storage sheds. But we know out of sight is out of mind as all those tools, storage containers, gadgets, and excess stuff you had to move out of the house become forgotten. Expensive monthly car payments and insurance pay for cars that end up parked in the driveway or on the street since there's no room in the garage. Latte, my car, was so happy when I finally got to park her in the garage, and I was so happy to close the garage door with her tucked safely inside, protected from the elements.

Most storage units are initially rented with good intentions but ultimately result in regret and resentment. Over the years, I've helped a few friends clean out their storage units. Some eventually release the rental unit, but they've all told me the same thing, *"I wish I had done this much earlier. I could have saved a ton of money."* By the time all the boxes were sifted and sorted, including items that had been damaged over time, very few things still held value. The rest was deemed junk or trash. Paying years' worth of monthly storage unit payments is an expensive way to store eventual junk and trash, not to mention all the time and energy asking friends and family to help move it around multiple times, only to end up dumping or donating it.

Less is truly more enlightening when it comes to "stuff." When we shed the clutter, clean the space, replace or repair our building and possessions, and beautify the space, we see our health improve, our money flow increase, our relationships bloom, and our happiness grow. Our palace is a reflection of who we are, how we believe we should be treated, and what we believe ourselves to be.

9

What's in Your Condiment Cabinet?

Herbs, Spices, Bone Broth, Financial, Recycle, Help Needed, and Everything Else

You mean, salt and pepper for your food? Yes, but there's more. Lots more. Just about every condiment or "thing" in your life can be evaluated, and most likely there is a more holistic way of making it work better toward your overall **wellness**.

The White Dangers: Salt, Sugar, and Flour

You can pretty much say "the white stuff" doesn't serve your overall health; however, there is always a healthier alternative.

Let's start with salt: NOT all salt is created equal. Do you believe that "salt is bad for you"? This cautionary statement is flawed and misleading because it does not specify the type of salt to stay away from. Conventional ionized table salt—the pretty, perfectly ground white substance that we see on many dining tables and restaurants—has been refined, stripped, and bleached of the natural nutrients the body needs to function. This is the type of salt to stay away from.

On the other hand, high mineral, nutrient rich Himalayan salt and sea salt, course-rock like salts and pink salts are untreated, unheated, and naturally dried. From unpolluted waters or salt caves they are transferred to evaporation ponds for drying. The result? Sparkling crystals containing essential trace minerals from our earth, natural streams, and oceans. These unrefined salts provide essential minerals needed for good health.

Lastly, don't get sticker shock. If you've been used to paying a dollar or two for your table salt, it's because of the lack of quality and sourcing. For a natural, high-quality salt, you may need to pay two or three times that. *You get what you pay for, and **You** are worth every dollar!*

The same goes with white **flour** which provides little nutrition, it's highly acidic, and can create digestive issues. Regular consumption of white flour can lead to conditions like a fatty liver and raises bad cholesterol in your bloodstream, resulting in several health issues such as high blood pressure, weight gain, mood swings, and progression toward obesity. Better choices include almond, coconut, oat, whole-meal or earthy-colored bread flours. For sandwich alternatives there are lettuce or cabbage wraps, or brown rice cakes. Try both! In your next sandwich consider using one bread slice and lettuce or cabbage on the other side.

Then there are the major discussions around

carbohydrates/gluten. I believe one should not cut them out completely, since meals without carbs can cause liver damage. It's all about the quantity and types of carbs you're eating. Multigrain and whole wheat bread can be part of a healthy and balanced eating plan, since they contain additional fiber and nutrition compared to their plain white counterpart.

We might have grown up eating white bread, which is why we *think* we like it, but it's quite bland. Whole wheat and multigrain varieties offer so much more in the way of texture and flavor. For added crunch, flavor, and nutrients you could choose a seeded loaf.

Let's not forget vegetables have "carbs" too. Of course, if there is an auto-immune or allergy concern, a gluten-free diet is appropriate. One of my favorite quick breakfast light meals is a slice of toasted Ezekiel brand bread with a mashed avocado spread, topped with pumpkin seeds, and a cup of unsweetened almond or coconut milk—delicious!

Sugar and Sweeteners

I saved the sweetener condiment for last of the trio, like dessert. **Sugar addiction is the root of many of our chemical and physical health problems.** Sugar comes in many forms, from many sources, and in many disguises like breads, soda pop, flavored waters, candy, fast food, dairy such as milk and yogurt, and packaged goods like cereals, oatmeal, granola bars, cookies, etc., most of which are damaging to our bodies and minds.

The worst sugars, in order, are:

Avoid	Healthier Selection
High fructose corn syrup	Raw organic honey
Aspartame, sucralose, and saccharin (blue, yellow, and pink packets)	Organic stevia
Agave	Raw maple syrup
White sugar	Organic brown or coconut sugar

Herbs

Herbs are nature's miracle workers. From cilantro, parsley, sage, rosemary, and oregano, to dill, basil, chamomile, horsetail, maca, and more; herbs are multi-purpose, multi-method little wonders for emotional, chemical, mental, physical, and spiritual health and healing. From hormonal imbalance to headaches, and gum infections to skin and hair conditions, and other ailments, herbs are powerful condiments and an absolute necessity for our pantries and wellness cabinets.

Spices

There are many spices available to enhance our food and satisfy even finicky pallets. Have fun and learn the benefits of these gems! One of the most beneficial of spices is turmeric. Turmeric is a root spice used in many Indian, Thai, and Ayurvedic recipes. Its properties are extremely helpful in supporting the liver function, reducing and preventing inflammation in the body, and increasing a sense of calmness in the central nervous system. Use this in tea, vegetable and bean dishes, and any dishes that you want an extra dash of spice and healing properties.

One of the most delicious and fun, as well as healing recipes is using turmeric in golden milk. Before bed, or sometime after dinner, or any time you want to rest and calm yourself, heat any milk alternative, such as coconut, almond, hemp, rice, cashew, or oat milk, then add a half teaspoon of organic honey or maple syrup, a teaspoon of turmeric, a quarter teaspoon of cinnamon, a dash of ginger, and a pinch of black or cayenne pepper (to activate the turmeric). Stir and let sit for a few minutes. Enjoy this delicious drink as well as build your immune system.

Here are just a few of my favorite herbs and spices and their benefits:

- Garlic: supports heart health and has antibacterial properties.
- Cinnamon: a powerful antioxidant that fights inflammation, lowers cholesterol, and balances blood sugar.
- Peppermint: improves headache pain and other associated symptoms of irritable bowel syndrome, or digestive issues and soothes nausea; increases energy.

- Cayenne: boosts metabolism and increases circulation (as do other hot peppers).

- Sage: improves memory and enhances brain function properties.

There is such an incredible variety of herbs and spices we can use to make each meal unique, super tasty, and nourishing all while building and strengthening our overall **Wellness**.

Minerals, Vitamins, and Supplements

Minerals are what the earth is made of. Minerals are what our bones, hair, skin, teeth, and tissues are made of. Because we suffer from low nutrient and polluted soil and water, mineral supplementation is a must for everyone. However, it's imperative to know why we suffer from mineral deficiency and what to do about it. Contrary to conventional advertising, dairy does not provide minerals that our bodies can really absorb. Our high animal protein diets have actually increased our fat levels and decreased our mineral and vitamin levels.

We have slowly evolved into a culture that consumes a highly processed, high animal protein, high sugar, high caffeine, high alcohol, and high prescription medication diet—and yet we consume little of the vitamin and mineral rich organic, plant-based foods and natural mineral spring water our bodies need.

The best source of minerals—that the body is able to fully

absorb—do not come from milk or cows, but from plants. Grown in earth's naturally mineralized soil, green leafy vegetables, herbs, spices, and fruits are the secret to re-mineralizing the body.

If you are wanting to increase your protein, understand that the body creates protein from the foods we eat, when our bodies are functioning at the capacity they were designed to. Rather than increasing animal protein intake, research how much protein the body actually needs. Use research from sources that are not funded by specific food (i.e. beef and dairy) industries. Use food sources of protein that are just as high, if not higher in protein levels than animal protein, and that our bodies can optimally digest, such as beans, legumes, nuts, and grains, such as quinoa.

If you are wanting to supplement your diet, the best products to use are those that are whole, organic, food-based supplements in forms that easily and quickly break down in our digestive processes. Hard pills and tablets do not break down quickly and, in fact, actually pass through our bodies only 10-25% broken down, with the remaining 75-90% eliminated almost intact by our bodies.

Bone Broth

The best form of animal protein and minerals is derived from bone broth. It has quickly become one of the most popular health-boosting additions over the last decade. Bone broth from beef, chicken, buffalo, and lamb is highly nutritious and healing for all kinds of ailments, including skin conditions, chronic fatigue, anemia, certain autoimmune conditions, and it boosts immune function and other health challenges. It's packed with nutrients, easy to digest, rich in flavor, and is loaded with restorative amino acids. Again, the quality of the bones will be important to the benefits gained.

Simple recipes to make bone broth include beef marrow and knuckle bones, plenty of filtered water, apple cider vinegar, sea salt, and vegetables such as onions, carrots, celery, parsley, etc. Cooking time can vary from 24-72 hours in a crockpot. Enjoy this nutritious drink/meal. The longer the cooking time, the greater the benefits.

MSG and Other Ingredients

When you are shopping for the condiments mentioned, including supplements, herbs, and spices, try to select organic, whole food-based versions and watch for hidden additives, such as MSG. Here are some excerpts from Dr. Mercola's website article, "A Story Called MSG: Is This Silent Killer Lurking in Your Kitchen Cabinets?"

- Monosodium glutamate (MSG) is a flavor enhancer added to thousands of foods that you and your family regularly eat. It's also one of the worst food additives on the market.

- MSG is an excitotoxin, which means that it overexcites your cells in a range from damage to death. It causes varying degrees of brain damage and is a potential trigger for worsening learning disabilities.

- Common adverse effects linked to regular consumption of MSG include obesity, eye damage, headaches, fatigue, disorientation, depression, rapid heartbeat, tingling, and numbness.

- Early studies suggested 25-30% of the US population was intolerant of MSG levels found in food. Today, an estimated 40% of the population may be impacted.

- In general, the more processed a food is, the higher the chance that it contains MSG, or other synthetic ingredients.

Watch out for ingredients such as "anti-clumping" agents, aluminum hydroxide, refined sugar, stearic acid, sodium ferrocyanide, calcium phosphate, and other additives.

Like everything else in today's consumer driven culture, you'll have a ton of choices, so read labels for added ingredients that do not serve your health, including "natural flavors," a phrase that sounds good but is actually carefully worded to disguise the fact they are unnecessary and unhealthy.

As you read earlier, there can be many toxins in our foods. As a Hispanic woman, and knowing that obesity and high blood pressure are prevalent in our culture, I want to point out a common toxin: MSG, found in many Hispanic households. In particular, it is in a very popular soup broth seasoning/enhancer. I was pleased to know that the maker of this Hispanic line has now rolled out a cleaner version without this toxin and I applaud any company's efforts in improving their products and making healthier versions.

It's important to read the labels and choose things without MSG and other ingredients you cannot pronounce.

So now we get into the "other" condiments of our lives, as mentioned at the beginning of the chapter.

Financial

While this book is primarily on health, why would I bring up finances? Again, it's part of having a "balanced life," which can give you improved health and happiness.

When your money matters are under control, you feel the peace and confidence behind your decisions. Unfortunately, many fall in the "broke" category for several reasons:

- extravagant or foolish spending

- lack of a budget or discipline to follow it

- poor stewardship

- simply lazy; unwilling to work; depending on others such as parents, government, etc.

- inability to change mental patterns (I grew up poor and will always be poor)

- not valuing money

- circumstances beyond control, unexpected illness,

loss of a primary job, death in the family

Recycle

Recycling is the process of converting waste materials into new materials and objects. Sounds like a no-brainer, but you would be surprised at how much is wasted, which contributes to the breaking down of our world's natural resources.

You probably are already doing some kind of recycling, and I encourage you to step it up some more to help preserve our wonderful planet. While doing so, you will feel good as "contributing" always adds happiness to our emotional fuel tank.

Holistic Chamber of Commerce (HCC)

What's this? Perhaps you think only individual cities have a Chamber of Commerce organization. Well, guess again! Just 10 years ago, Camille Leon founded this great organization to help those wanting access to **holistic** practitioners to assist them in their journey.

There are now 35 chapters nationwide to help you find partners that can aid you in this path. Since the birth of the Orange County chapter formed by Jan Edwards, I have been a member of this resourceful organization:

www.holisticchamberofcommerce.com

Help Needed

Like many people, I've read a ton of books over the years on health promising secrets to change your life. And they could, if you are mentally ready to commit. Like I said earlier in the book, this is no quick fix if you want lasting results. I found that getting help from a group program, a wellness coach, a nutritionist, or other professional will make your commitment a higher possibility of reality. It is truly my desire and prayer that this book inspired you enough to keep that commitment to yourself, once and for all.

10

Why Does Spirituality Heal?

Do you remember back in Chapter 1 where I said that one of the most important steps on your path to wellness is to answer the question about being well versus unwell? If you skipped that part, or didn't complete it all the way, stop reading Chapter 10 right now. Put a bookmark on this page, go back to Chapter 1, and complete those questions. *If you did complete those questions in Chapter 1,* you are ready for the second most important step on your path to wellness.

What? Why have I waited to share the second most important step on your path to wellness until almost the end of the book? Reading this step at the end of the book will leave you with a lasting impact that will drastically change your health—*and your life*—for the better, *forever.*

If you're like me, you were raised as, or later became, a follower of Catholicism or Christianity. Or, maybe it was Buddhism, Hinduism, Islam, or one of the other 10,000 religions of the world. Perhaps you didn't grow up with any religion, or you just prefer to call yourself spiritual. You may be agnostic or atheist. Rest assured, I'm not about to go into a religious sermon or debate, and I am not judging anyone for their beliefs. I just want to share something very personal that not only changed my well-being, but unexpectedly changed my heart and the very foundation of my life.

In the years that I've been writing this book, my spirituality has drastically changed. In being born and raised Catholic, I knew nothing but those teachings. I didn't ask questions; just did what I was told. When Sunday came, we did not miss church, and we wore our "Sunday best." It was the norm to help others, be kind to others, serve others, and give to others. The religious practice was beautiful and reverent, and it served me well for those years.

I also remember dozens of repetitive prayers; yet, rarely looked inside the Bible. I didn't even own a Bible. I didn't see people walk into church with a Bible, except the priest who read scripture from it. At one point, I thought I was becoming a better person by praying one decade of the rosary (10+ prayers) every morning and would end up falling asleep. I just wasn't feeling the connection.

Going to church was an obligation. We were told that it was the right thing to do, regardless of whether we fell asleep during mass. We still had to go, to set an example. I am not putting down Catholicism, or any religion, but for me it didn't feel complete, as I wasn't deepening spiritually or developing a heartfelt relationship. Regardless, the Catholic church will always have a very special place in my heart and I feel the reverence when I occasionally visit.

About 10 years ago, I started attending a private Bible study led by a wonderful Catholic woman. The first day I walked in, I felt embraced by her and a wonderful group primarily made up of Catholics, one Protestant, and I think one Christian. They all had one common goal: to learn more about Jesus Christ. It was really the first time in my life that I felt inclined to open, read, and understand the Bible. It wasn't easy, but I kept at it.

Initially, I didn't really understand three quarters of what I read. But as I studied the Bible more, and as I listened to pastors like Greg Laurie, Chuck Smith, Rick Warren, and David Jeremiah, *I felt a calling to connect directly with God* and the Bible for guidance, protection, and wisdom.

As I prayed directly to God and asked Him to help me really understand, it clicked. I became excited, and I began feeling the Holy Spirit in me.

It's hard to describe what that feels like, but it's an inner feeling. It's listening to my inner self. It didn't happen in one day or with one "aha moment." On the contrary, I have had a bazillion aha moments, and more and more of them have added to that feeling within me.

The change led to a completely different experience for me, but I wouldn't really call it a change. It was a drastic **transformation** of my mind and of my heart. It was so amazingly incredible! What a huge difference it was from the religious doctrine and repetitive practices I had been following for almost 50 years. I felt the change move from my head to my heart. That's what I would describe is the difference between religion and spirituality. Religion is being more in the head. Spirituality is being more in the heart.

Heart

When I began having a personal relationship with God in my heart and allowed the Holy Spirit to live in my heart, I experienced the ultimate transformation—being happier with who I am and becoming a better human being. Having this spiritual connection has played a huge role in my wanting to better myself, take care of this body temple that He gave me for my time here, and love myself more.

As I write this, we just passed Valentine's Day 2022, one year from the day I was baptized as a Christian and accepted Jesus as my Savior. I intentionally chose that day because I really believe in love, and I knew that day would be very special for me to remember.

So, what does all of this have to do with healing?

Forgiveness

Love is the most powerful healer. By opening my heart for a direct relationship with God and loving myself more, I was able to have enough love and compassion to forgive those who hurt me. As human beings, we will be hurt by one or many people in our lifetimes, whether intentional or not. If we don't forgive, we create a barrier in our ability to move forward in life. While we may put the hurt aside or think we have buried it, it keeps resurfacing. It haunts us.

For many people, overeating, having food addictions, and even not eating are rooted in their experiences of being hurt by people during their childhood. If the wound isn't healed with the proper love and care, it will keep reopening. It will continue in one way or another. And it's going to hurt, again and again and again, unless we embrace forgiveness.

Once a wound is healed, meaning that we have decided to feel love, not resentment, and forgive the person who hurt us, we naturally stop thinking about it. We stop feeling the pain. We start truly moving on.

Forgiving doesn't mean we have to forget because there is no magic pill we can take to forget something. But we have to deal with the wound. We have to learn how to sincerely forgive. Most important of all, we have to love ourselves enough to forgive ourselves. No sin is big enough that God cannot forgive, if you truly repent.

The Lord's Prayer, the main prayer in every Bible, says, *"Forgive us, as we forgive others."*

Forgiveness is a huge piece of true and complete healing. If I had not been able to forgive the people who hurt me the most, I don't think I would be compelled to want to finish this book. I would not have such a passion to share this with so many people. When I get in front of people, I can really feel the influence I'm having on their thinking and their belief that they can change their health.

I thank God for gifting me with that motivation, that inspiration.

Helping Others

Another piece of spirituality that has played an even bigger part of healing my life is what I like to refer to as "Pay It Forward," one of the components of the WOW! Program. I have such joy in doing projects that help others by paying it forward. It's like turning around as you climb the hill and putting your hand out to help someone else get up the hill. It's not about who's further ahead or who's winning or losing. It's not a race. It's not about the bigger car or the better this or that. It's not a competition. And, it's not about keeping up with the Joneses. It's about helping someone else go on the journey with you. It's about giving a helping hand. Helping others is such a beautiful thing.

Helping others is being the image of Jesus. He always helped people, including those with leprosy who no one wanted to touch or have anything to do with. Rather than want to stay away from them or put them away, Jesus was not afraid to touch them. That's how we should try to see people, even the homeless. Who's to know why they're homeless. Some love it. Some don't know anything else. Others just need a little compassion and help to restore their lives.

A Personal Relationship

People often think, *Oh, Christians think they have a perfect life. Because they know God, they're always going to be happy and everything's going to be perfect.* That is far from the truth. The Bible says that we're going to have tribulations, and we're going to suffer. The level of suffering will always be different for every person, but the degree that we are willing to open ourselves to love, to forgive, to feel the Holy Spirit, and to help others directly affects the severity and duration of our suffering.

Even in the midst of difficulty, we can live with confidence because the Spirit of the living God enables us to. And even in this world that is so full of fear, distrust, and uncertainty, please don't allow yourself to be influenced by the negative messages—just keep your eyes on Christ. Facing each day with His strength will drive away or lessen the doubt and anxiety. One of His promises is that He will never leave us or forsake us. By His grace, He has forgiven us, and if we are walking in His path we will have heaven and brighter times to look forward to.

The result of my personal transformation is my inner knowing that I have a stable and reliable relationship with the One who will fulfill His promises to lead and guide me. I know that every promise He has made is going to fulfill me.

Not all of my transformation has been easy. Much time and devotion has created the space that I am now in, and I am loving it. We have perfect and beautiful days, and we have dark and down days. What I now have in my spirit helps me to go through the dark and down days and moments, rather than discard or ignore them, and arrive back at a better place sooner than before. And that is what has healed me; having that inner strength to recognize that I have a Higher Being that is with me. We can be *in* the world, but we don't have to be *of* the world.

Embracing spirituality in your heart may be difficult at first, but what good thing in your life was easy to acquire? As anxiety rises with everything going on, we've got a narrow, steep path ahead of us. Having a pronounced spiritual relationship in our hearts lights up our paths, comforts us on our journeys, and heals our body, mind, and spirit.

Where to Begin

Healing the spirit is not a one step process, just like wellness is not a one pill or one exercise commitment. It's an everyday development that grows with baby steps. Someone's baby steps may seem like mammoth steps for you, or vice versa. But the first step is deciding, *I want to have a more joyful life. I want to have more hope. I want to better myself. I want to take care of this temple that I've been given.*

Once you've made the decision to begin or continue your healing transformation, visit a few Bible based churches or communities and join one that you feel the Holy Spirit in.

One of my favorite parts of church is having communion. Putting the wafer in my mouth symbolized having a piece of God in me, with me. It was the thing that gave me a feeling of connection with Him. I was communing with Him. The WOW! Program has been successful because of its community.

We naturally need connection and interaction with others. So many people are depressed in these times because they've had to work from home, or stay home away from others. With the Covid situation, many people have become depressed. There are some who thrive in being by themselves, but even they are re-energized when they are connecting with others in a warm, caring group gathering. We need hugs. We need physical interaction, touch, heart connection, and spiritual communion. Babies who are not held, nuzzled, and hugged enough can stop growing and even die. Virtual meetings don't always fulfill our basic needs. We're human *beings*. We're meant to *be with* and commune with other human beings. Healing the heart and spirit can only happen when we're in the presence of others, sharing our hearts.

The Ultimate Healing

Happiness is temporary. It comes and it goes because it's dependent on an external condition or person. JOY, on the other hand, comes from *within* us, not outside of us. We get joy from our heart relationship with a Higher Being, from forgiving, from loving, and from helping others. Joy helps us look forward, not only in the day to day and tomorrow, but beyond this life experience. When you can walk through even the dark days and feel the seed of joy still present inside of you, knowing it's always there, that's when you know you are truly healing on the inside.

Do you see now why I believe Spiritual Healing is the second most important step on your path to wellness, and why I saved it until the end of the book? I hope that my words and personal experience has not left you feeling judged for wherever you are or aren't in your spiritual journey. I hope, instead, that I have motivated your mind and inspired your heart to include your own spiritual healing in your healthy lifestyle changes. I guarantee you will be surprised at the impact it has on your well-being—*and your life*. Who knows? It may even lead to your own profound Transformation. ***If not now, WHEN?***

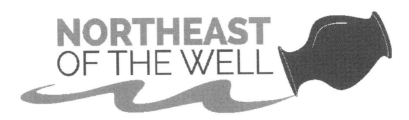

Thank you for contributing! Ten percent (10%) of the profit from the sale of this book will go to a certified 501(c)(3) non-profit organization dedicated to helping broken humans restore their faith and dignity locally in Orange County. This organization was founded by Laura Johnson-Suk in 2011.

They are a church on the go as they bring God's Word into places of desperate need, with a focus on those in recovery and restoration. As a Christian ministry, they strive to bring light into hard places: county programs, transitional living homes, shelters, safe houses, jails, etc. Seventy-five percent (75%) of those they serve come from families where chronic addiction, incarceration, abuse, and poverty go back two or more generations. Most have been through trauma such as sexual exploitation and human trafficking.

Their vision is simple: *the outcast becomes the witness.*

Northeast of the Well
2025 Newport Blvd., Suite # 110
Costa Mesa, CA 92627
949-515-WELL (9355)
www.northeastofthewell.org

Acknowledgment of great Professionals who in some special way, through their individual help or their business, have had a positive impact in my health life (not in any specific order):

Dr. Marshall E. Reddick, PhD
Real Estate Investor / Longevity Educator
Happily Enjoying Retirement

Dr. Linda Marquez Goodine, CN, DC
Holistic Wellness, Chiropractor, Speaker, Author
PremierHealthOC.com

Ms. Ivy Irvine Bridge
Iridologist aka "The Colon Queen"
Ivys.com

Steven Bridge
Operations Manager
Ivys.com

Joshua Rosenthal
Founder / Director
IntegrativeNutritionInstitute.com

Dr. Pedram Shojai
Health Educator, Movie Maker, Author, Speaker
Well.org

Dr. Billy DeMoss
Chiropractor, CalJam Founder, Wellness Enthusiast
DemossChiropractic.com

Gerry Warkentine
Bible Study Leader
EstherWomanofFaith.com

Arnoux Goran
Health Enthusiast
TotalHealthMasteryUSA.com

Drs. Marcus and Elizabeth Plourde
Electromagnetic Field Educators / Radiation Protection Devices
EmfFreedom.com

Dr. Paul Petty, DC
Chiropractor, Bowen Therapist
Petty-Chiropractic.com

Jan Edwards
Business Consultant
Founder, OC Chapter, Holistic CofC
InspiredLifeGuide.com

Edward J. Synicky
Financial Advisor
Happily Enjoying Retirement

Camille Leon
Founder, Holistic CofC
HolisticChamberofCommerce.com

Ruben Mata
Motivator, Speaker, Author
RubenMata.com

Reggie Adelaars
Young Living Essential Oils Consultant and Raindrop
Technique Specialist
Health4HisGlory.com

Linda Gravani
Business Advisor
President, Lake Balboa Neighborhood Council

Omar Ramirez
Computer Xpert
xirtam_edoc@hotmail.com

Patricia Garza Pinto
Holistic Health and Wellness Practitioner
DivineMountainRetreat.com

Suzanne Bordbar
Graphics Designer
Susanne.Bordbar@gmail.com

Trina Harris
Iridologist, Herbalist
TreeofNaturalHealth@yahoo.com

Eva Corona
Hairdresser / Our First Wow! Program Location
Emmanuel Hair Salon

Frances Pullin
President, Tustin Chapter, Holistic CofC
FrancesPullin.com

Christopher Bissonnette
V.P., Tustin Chapter, Holistic CofC
ChrisBissonnette.com

Cindy Hodgkins
Wow! Graduate / Salvationist
SalvationArmyusa.org

Lesli Remington
Certified Clinical Thermographer
ThermalBodyScans.com

Mitzi Cristobal
Cooking Demos / Titanium Cookware for Improved Health
HappyCookingCo.com

Sharon Barnard
Holy Yoga Instructor
InhaleLoveYoga.com

Erik Sahakian
Publisher
AbundantHarvestPublishing.com

About the Author

Lupe Silva was born in Sahuayo, Michoacán, Mexico in 1963 and three months later, her family moved to the US.

Throughout her childhood, Lupe struggled with obesity and continued into adulthood with many ailments, including major depression.

While her initial studies were in Human Resources, with a concentration in Benefits, she found herself gravitating toward helping others successfully improve their health.

However, her own health and happiness had reached "rock bottom," until she received an answer to prayer. After a 20-plus-year career, Lupe realized that corporate work was not a path she wanted to continue and redirected her focus to natural health.

Her personal healing journey made her passionate about sharing her healing success secrets with others. Following formal training from IIN (Institute for Integrative Nutrition), the world's largest holistic nutrition school, Lupe became a certified Health Coach.

Integrating her independent studies and experiences into her work, she came to the realization that natural body, mind and spirit health and healing were the remedy for many challenges and overall wellness. With new clarity, Lupe launched her current business in 2015, *Wellness Path*.

Included is *The WOW! Program* (Working on Wellness), an onsite group program for transforming tired, overweight, or health challenged individuals into healthier and motivated team members. *The WOW! Program* helps companies maximize employee productivity by introducing and guiding participants to incorporate holistic principles of healthy living, thereby increasing the health, energy, productivity, disease prevention, and quality of life for their employees. Her program is also available for residential and church communities.

Lupe Silva has served on the leadership team of the Holistic Chamber of Commerce, Tustin Chapter (initially named, Orange County) since 2011 and many pay-it-forward projects. Her deepest desire has become her signature trademark: leaving a positive impact on the lives of the people she meets—*in particular, the Latino community*—and providing awareness and support for motivating an intrinsic drive for healthy personal lifestyle changes.

Happily married for 38 years, with two grown sons and four furry grandkids, Lupe and her husband reside in Orange County, California.

For information and participation in *The Wow! Program*, or to request Lupe Silva to speak at your company meeting on wellness lifestyle, please contact **info@wellnesspath.us.**

www.WellnessPath.us